Magnetic Resonance Imaging and Computed Tomography

Clinical Neuro-Orbital Anatomy

Jonathan D. Wirtschafter, MD

Department of Ophthalmology
University of Minnesota

Eric L. Berman, MD

Department of Ophthalmology
University of Rochester

Carolyn S. McDonald, MD

Ulster CT Medical Associates
Kingston, New York

AMERICAN ACADEMY OF OPHTHALMOLOGY

American Academy of Ophthalmology

655 Beach Street

P.O. Box 7424

San Francisco, CA 94120-7424

OPHTHALMOLOGY MONOGRAPHS COMMITTEE

C. P. Wilkinson, MD, Chairperson
Barrett G. Haik, MD
Harold E. Shaw, Jr, MD

ACADEMY STAFF

Kathryn A. Hecht, EdD
Director of Education

Hal Straus
Managing Editor, Ophthalmology Monographs

Pearl C. Vapnek
Medical Editor

Design and Production
Christy Butterfield Design

Illustrations
Barbara Barnett

Copyright © 1992 American Academy of Ophthalmology®
All rights reserved.

Library of Congress Cataloging-in-Publication Data

Wirtschafter, Jonathan Dine, 1935–
    Magnetic resonance imaging and computed tomography : clinical
neuro-orbital anatomy / Jonathan D. Wirtschafter, Eric L. Berman,
Carolyn S. McDonald.
       p.   cm.
    An expansion of: Computed tomography / by Jonathan D. Wirtschafter
and Saul Taylor. c1982.
    Includes bibliographical references and index.
    ISBN 1-56055-010-4
    1. Eye—Magnetic resonance imaging—Atlases.   2. Eye—Tomography—
Atlases.   3. Visual pathways—Magnetic resonance imaging—Atlases.
4. Visual pathways—Tomography—Atlases.   I. Berman, Eric L.
II. McDonald, Carolyn S.   III. Wirtschafter, Jonathan Dine, 1935–   .
IV. Title.
    [DNLM: 1. Eye—anatomy & histology—atlases.   2. Eye Diseases—
diagnosis—atlases.   3. Magnetic Resonance Imaging—methods—
atlases.   4. Tomography, X-Ray Computed—methods—atlases.
W1 OP372L v.6 / WW 17 W799m]
QM511.W55   1992
617.7′1548—dc20
DNLM/DLC
for Library of Congress   92-49178
                                                              CIP

Printed in Singapore through Palace Press San Francisco.

Contents

FEB 2 6 1996 c.1 acu $65.90

Preface

Neuro-orbital imaging using computed tomography (CT) and magnetic resonance imaging (MRI) has revolutionized the practice of neuro-ophthalmology. The introduction of CT in 1972 permitted ophthalmologists to become aware of clinically important anatomic relationships that had not been visualized previously. More recently, clinical MRI has become widely available and continues to undergo technical improvement, increasing the amount and quality of diagnostic information yielded the clinician. Compared with conventional x-ray films, CT scanning greatly improves the information content because it allows evaluation of both the soft tissues and the bony orbit, as well as the brain. Conventional x-ray films are useful in assessing the skull and in locating metallic foreign bodies, as well as providing information about soft tissue where natural contrast is present, such as the presence of orbital soft tissues in the air-filled maxillary sinus.

In most circumstances, MRI offers clear advantages over CT by providing better definition of not only tissues but also circulating and stationary fluids. MRI scanning further enhances the information obtained because it allows delineation between white matter and gray matter, as well as providing midline sagittal imaging, which is not accessible with CT, and identifying edema. In addition, MRI permits angiographic studies without intravenous contrast agents and spares the patient the dangers of irradiation. In many respects, the two modalities (MRI and CT) are complementary, providing useful comparison studies. To better understand anatomic relationships, ophthalmologists should become familiar with the information provided by both types of imaging.

This atlas of correlative neuro-orbital anatomy reflects the maturation and wide availability of MRI technology. Thus, while the book includes both MRI and CT images of most regions, not all possible CT images of the brain are represented, particularly scans within the posterior fossa, where the lack of soft tissue detail and the artifact created by bony structures produce images that compare unfavorably to those produced with MRI. CT images are preferred where they provide bony details not equaled by MRI (ie, bony foramina) and contribute to the knowledge of paranasal sinus anatomy, which has become more important to ophthalmologists since the development of endoscopic sinus surgical techniques.

As this monograph was in preparation, a new generation of MR scanners was being introduced. These machines, called *gradient scanners*, will enable the production of images in milliseconds that currently require minutes. These new units should allow increased resolution with decreased movement artifact because of the reduced imaging time. However, the safety of these scanners has yet to be fully evaluated.

Chapter 1 of this monograph is intended to provide a non-mathematical introduction to the physics and techniques of imaging. The main body of the atlas, Chapters 2 through 7, is not intended to be a comprehensive text concerning radiology of the eye, orbit, or nervous system. Nor is it a textbook of pathologic radiologic findings seen in various disease entities. Numerous excellent reference sources are presently available for both these purposes. Those images demonstrating pathology that are included are intended only to assist in identifying relevant anatomic structures. For many structures, information is provided concerning normal anatomic relationships and the resulting pathologic significance. The index is designed to save the reader time by pointing out the plane in which a given structure is shown in each figure.

We hope that this monograph will enable ophthalmologists to identify anatomic structures of clinical concern so that they will be more specific when ordering CT and MRI studies and will be better able to interpret the scans. Our view is that ophthalmologists should review the scans of their own patients, to assess whether the requested studies were done and whether they properly demonstrate the relevant structures. For example, if orbital scans are requested and 6-mm-thick slices of the brain are obtained, the structure of interest may be missed. Good communication between the requesting physician and the neuroradiologist is essential in obtaining useful studies.

We wish to acknowledge specifically our appreciation of the efforts of many persons who contributed to this monograph, and particularly our editor, Ms Pearl C. Vapnek. Gratitude is extended to Anne G. Osborn, MD, and Carl B. Tubbs, MD, for providing certain MR images used in this atlas. Benjamin C. P. Lee, MD, supplied the MR angiograms, and Saul Taylor, MD, provided the majority of the CT images. We would also like to acknowledge the efforts of Mr Ralph Fernandez and his staff in the Biomedical Graphics Department at the University of Minnesota in producing the excellent-quality prints of the images. This process involved rephotographing and reprinting several images to provide necessary detail of specific structures. The Department of Radiology at the University of Minnesota generously contributed MRI scanner time and personnel.

Preparation of this volume was facilitated, in part, by gifts from Mr Donald Gabbert and Mrs Louise Gabbert, Mr Glen Taylor and Mrs Katharine Burch Taylor, and the Frank E. Burch, MD, Endowed Professorship of Ophthalmology at the University of Minnesota.

Jonathan D. Wirtschafter, MD
Eric L. Berman, MD
Carolyn S. McDonald, MD

Fundamentals of MRI and CT Scanning

Although this monograph is primarily concerned with imaging, identification, and clinical significance, this chapter has been included to provide some basic explanations of the technology involved in MRI (magnetic resonance imaging) and CT (computed tomography) scanning of the neuro-orbital system in health and disease. For more details concerning the physics of MRI and CT, the reader is advised to consult the many excellent imaging texts, some of which are listed at the end of this chapter.

1-1

MAGNETIC RESONANCE IMAGING

The demonstration of human anatomy using the techniques of magnetic resonance was first accomplished by a team at the University of Nottingham in 1976. This accomplishment rests on a broadly based body of knowledge and techniques that encompasses much of modern physics. The scientific foundation involves notions of atomic and molecular structure and the concept of nuclear magnetic resonance. First observed in the late 1940s, the actual phenomenon of nuclear magnetic resonance could be produced in uniform, bulk materials contained in test tubes or similar chambers. In 1973, P. G. Lauterbur suggested that magnetic field gradients could encode position-dependent imaging information. This was an opportune time, as computed tomography was just coming into clinical practice. Although magnetic resonance imaging is conceptually and technically much more complex than x-ray computed tomographic imaging, the speed of progress has been remarkable. Magnetic resonance imaging evolved rapidly

with the increased availability of high-field-strength magnets for stimulating the magnetic resonance phenomenon and of many computer programs for analyzing the images and controlling the magnetic devices. The technique of MRI can still be regarded as being in a rapid phase of evolution, whereas CT seems to have reached a plateau where its technologic limits may have already been achieved.

1-1-1 Physical Principles

Despite the technical complexity of MRI, ophthalmologists will be encouraged to know that the physics of magnetic resonance can be more easily understood by emphasizing models that are analogous to those used for explaining the physics of light. Some phenomena of light can best be described by classical wave theory while other phenomena of light are best illustrated by quantum particle theory, even though the two approaches may have apparent contradictions. Similarly, the physics of MRI can sometimes best be understood with a quantum-mechanical model, in which each proton can be in either one of two states (parallel or anti-parallel), or with a classical mechanical model, in which the net magnetic moment vector of all protons can be located with regard to a three-dimensional frame of reference. This three-dimensional frame of reference may be considered either as stationary, with its z axis coincident with that of the main (static) magnetic field, or as rotating, with its z axis coincident with the net magnetic vectors (M) produced by the precessing protons.

MRI is based on the principle that the nuclei of certain atoms become polarized or aligned (display magnetic moments) when placed in a static magnetic field (Figure 1-1). This magnetic property is

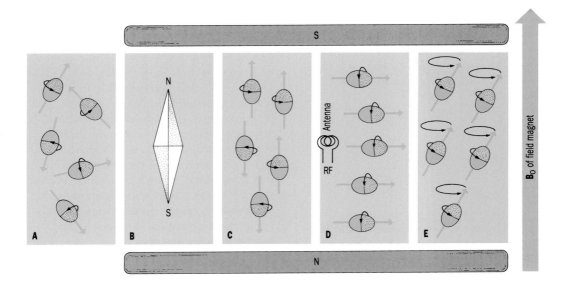

Figure 1-1 *Comparison of the magnetic properties of a compass with the magnetic resonance behavior of protons in several states. (A) No magnet: in the absence of a magnetic field, the protons are randomly aligned. (B) Compass needle in magnetic field: the compass needle aligns with the magnet but can point in only one direction.*
(C) In main magnetic field: the magnetized protons are "flipped" to align with the magnetic field, B_0, but may align parallel or antiparallel to the applied magnetic field. More protons align with the field than against it. The possibility of two orientations for the protons differs from the one orientation allowed for the compass needle.
(D) Immediately after application of a 90° RF pulse: the imposition of a 90° RF pulse by an antenna (diagrammed as a coil) causes all the protons that contributed to the net magnetic vector to flip in one direction in the transverse plane, where they all precess in phase. (E) Partial longitudinal relaxation and precession: after the end of a 90° RF burst, the protons relax toward the longitudinal axis and are seen precessing around that axis. A similar result occurs when the RF pulse is shorter than a pulse required for a 90° displacement. Such a pulse is said to tilt *the protons and is used in various imaging sequences.*

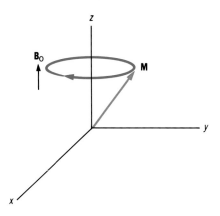

Figure 1-2 *The nuclear magnetization vector* **M** *rotates at the Larmor frequency around the main magnetic field vector* **B₀**, *which is defined as oriented in the z axis.* **M** *rotates in the clockwise direction (from y to x) as viewed from above at the Larmor frequency. The MRI signal obtained from the protons in each voxel must be detected and processed to obtain useful information.*

present only if the nucleus contains an odd number of nucleons (the sum of protons and neutrons). In particular, it is the odd number of protons in the nuclei of hydrogen (^{1}H), sodium (^{23}Na), and phosphorus (^{31}P) that is responsible for the magnetic moments in human tissues. This realignment is a statistical phenomenon, for not all nuclei will be equally realigned. When the magnetic field (designated as B_0) is activated, all of the atomic nuclei will be affected. However, a much smaller fraction of the nuclei will align against B_0 than with it, creating a net magnetic vector in the longitudinal direction of the magnetic field, designated the z axis (Figure 1-2). The behavior of hydrogen nuclei (protons) in a magnetic field can be compared and contrasted to that of a compass. The compass needle always points in one direction, but protons can align either parallel or antiparallel to the magnetic field. The protons aligned in the parallel direction are at a lower energy level than those aligned in the antiparallel direction. A quantum of energy must be absorbed by a proton oriented in the parallel direction for it to be transformed into a proton oriented in the antiparallel direction. Conversely, a proton oriented in the antiparallel direction must lose a quantum of energy to be transformed to a parallel orientation.

Transformations between parallel and antiparallel orientations can occur if the proton gains or emits energy by gaining or emitting one photon (as an RF wave) of the correct energy. Moreover, a proton in an antiparallel orientation can be struck by one photon and emit two photons, resulting in an energy loss sufficient to transform the proton to a parallel orientation. Low-strength magnets cause nearly equal numbers of protons to align in each direction; but as the magnetic field strength is increased, the magnetic dipoles of the individual protons tend to align in the lowest energy state parallel to the main magnetic field. This creates a net magnetic vector parallel to the direction of the magnet.

For each isotope that possesses a nuclear magnetic moment (eg, ^1H or ^{31}P), there is a characteristic resonant frequency (Larmor frequency) at which it absorbs energy. The Larmor frequency is related to intrinsic properties of that element and the strength of the static magnetic field (measured in tesla, abbreviated T). Thus, application of a radiofrequency wave of resonant frequency equal to the Larmor frequency provides the energy that will produce a realignment of the magnetic vector. This energy is re-emitted from the protons over time through a process known as *relaxation*. During relaxation, the torque of the static magnetic field exerted on the magnetic moment of the protons causes them to exhibit a type of movement called *precession:* the protons behave like small tops spinning around the axis of the magnetic field vector (see Figure 1-1). We are familiar with the force of gravity that causes the precession of a spinning top or gyroscope; when the device falls over, relaxation is completed. In the case of MRI, the magnetic force causes complete relaxation when all of the protons are realigned. Relaxation is the process whereby the absorbed energy is redistributed among the aligned protons (there is also some loss to the neighboring nuclei). Relaxation releases energy at the Larmor frequency and this energy can be detected with an antenna, often the same antenna that was used to excite the protons.

1-1-2 Extraction of Spatial Information

Once the protons are in an aligned equilibrium orientation, it becomes possible to use a burst of electromagnetic energy to manipulate the protons and produce clinically useful information. The imposition of the main magnetic field is somewhat analogous to installing the strings on a musical instrument and then applying tension to them (tuning). The tuning is accomplished by the gradient magnetic field. The plucking of the proton "strings" is done with a short pulse or burst of radiofrequency (RF) whose magnetic field is perpendicular to the static magnetic field. This RF pulse provides energy that is absorbed by the protons and brings them to a more excited state that changes the direction of their magnetic vectors. The length of the pulse can be varied to control the degree of change in the magnetic vector. The RF bursts can be designated as 90° or 180° pulses. The resultant movements of the protons can be called *flips* or *tilts* (see Figure 1-1). When the net magnetic vector is flipped 90° to the longitudinal axis (z), it is located in the transverse (x,y) plane.

In current clinical practice, only protons are used to produce MRI scans, because protons are abundant and their signal is easily detected. Most of the energy re-emitted by the protons in the tissue is absorbed within the tissue, but a small fraction of the energy is absorbed by the antenna receiver coil. The detected signal is proportional to the spin density: the number of nuclear magnetic moments per unit volume. The signal is received by an an-

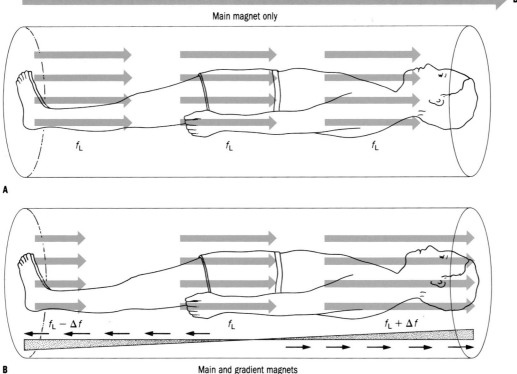

A Main magnet only

B Main and gradient magnets

B_0

f_L f_L f_L

$f_L - \Delta f$ f_L $f_L + \Delta f$

Figure 1-3 *Gradient magnets can alter the local magnetic field strength (represented by arrow length) from the uniform strength imposed by the main magnet (A). When the gradient magnet field is superimposed (B), unequal field strength results. Although the progression is continuous throughout the magnetic field, the strength in only three regions is shown for simplicity. Without the gradient magnets, the resonance frequency (f) is also uniform throughout the volume, but f changes (Δf) due to the gradient. The extent of the magnetic gradient is called its* bandwidth. *The gradient magnet tunes the system for the extraction of spatial information. For example, only the slice containing the head would be selected by an RF pulse of $f_L + \Delta f$. (f_L = Larmor frequency induced by main magnet)*

tenna arranged to detect precession of the magnetic dipole of protons only while they remain aligned in the transverse plane. If a signal were recorded as described above, it would be described as a measurement of free induction decay (FID). The longitudinal decay of each proton within the slice is somewhat analogous to that of each atom within a volume of unstable isotopes of one element, in that it behaves independently with its own timing. FID signals are not used clinically because their half-lives are not sufficiently long to allow the application of gradients necessary for localizing the signals in human patients. The pulse sequences that

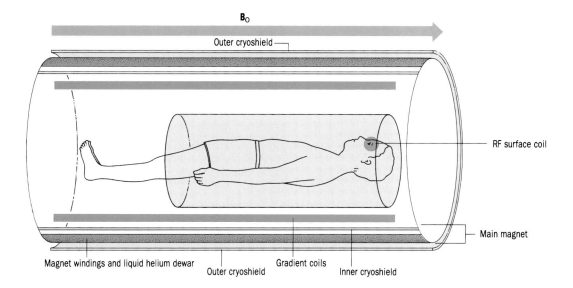

B_O

Outer cryoshield

RF surface coil

Main magnet

Magnet windings and liquid helium dewar

Outer cryoshield

Gradient coils

Inner cryoshield

are used to produce clinically useful signals are discussed in Section 1-1-4. The emitted signals are transformed by the computer into an image by a mathematical process called *two-* or *three-dimensional Fourier transformation.* This produces the familiar pictures seen on the printed films.

Nuclear magnetic resonance was initially a technique applied to small volumes of homogeneous chemicals in a vessel within homogeneous magnetic fields. To provide useful clinical information about the inhomogeneous environments of protons within a tissue space such as the skull or orbit, it is necessary to arrange for the selective excitation of a slice of tissue with an MRI scanning device. To accomplish this, a weak inhomogeneous gradient static magnetic field is superimposed on the strong homogeneous static magnetic field supplied by the main magnet (Figure 1-3). The weak magnetic field is produced by one or more accessory magnets called *gradient coils* (Figure 1-4). Three gradient

Figure 1-4 *Magnetic resonance scanning device, demonstrating the main magnet, gradient (magnet) coils, and RF surface coils. The use of surface coils is optional.* B_0, *the magnetic vector of the main magnet, is in the longitudinal plane (z axis) and is shown above the device. The transverse plane (x,y axes) is perpendicular to the longitudinal axis.*

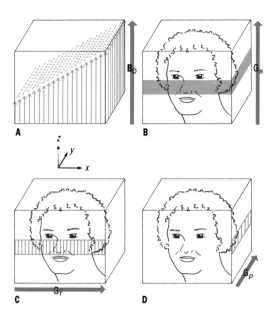

$$z \quad y \quad x$$

Figure 1-5 *Acquisition of a single-slice, two-dimensional Fourier transform image. (A) The gradients of the magnetic field strengths within the scanned volume produced by the main and gradient magnets. The direction of the B_0 arrow indicates the main magnetic field. The direction of increasing phase difference and increasing frequency within the slice is indicated by the arrows. (B) The dark volume is that excited by the RF pulses within the selected frequency range: the wider the range, the greater the slice thickness. This parameter is also designated as G_s, the slice-selection gradient. (C) The frequency-encoding gradient (G_f) is shown arbitrarily along the y axis of the transverse plane. (D) The phase-encoding gradient (G_p) is shown arbitrarily along the x axis of the transverse plane. Spatial localization within three-dimensional volumes (voxels) can be defined by the application of these gradients. The application of the x gradient while detecting the MRI signal assigns a unique frequency to each voxel according to its x coordinates. The application of a y gradient for a short period before the detection of the MRI signal assigns a unique phase to each voxel according to its y coordinates.*

coils are required to set up a three-dimensional imaging system.

A spatial coordinate system can be established that permits imaging of the axial, coronal, and sagittal orthogonal planes as well as oblique planes. Manipulating the gradient fields through orthogonal planes provides data for Fourier transformation and spatial reconstruction. This can be done by periodically adding y and z gradient fields to the static x gradient field.

The ability to directly obtain information in the midsagittal plane of the skull is one of the principal advantages of MRI over CT. Once the x, y, and z gradients have been established, a change of the exciting radiofrequency is the only requirement for changing which of the parallel planes is being imaged. The thickness of the parallel planes (slice thickness) is controlled by the bandwidth of the radiofrequency (Figure 1-5).

The MRI device contains RF receiver coils, which pick up the MRI signal that will later be amplified and analyzed. Although RF receiver coils are built into the scanner, they can be temporarily disconnected and replaced by smaller coils applied directly to parts of the body surface such as the orbit. Direct application improves the signal-to-noise (S/N) ratio and thus provides even greater resolution. Surface coils such as head and orbit coils have specific uses for evaluating the orbit and visual system. No matter where the receiver coils are placed, the only useful signal that can be detected is in the x,y plane, because the dominant magnetic field arises from the main bore magnet, the location of which is fixed.

Selective excitation of protons within a single slice will result when the precession frequency of the protons within the slice

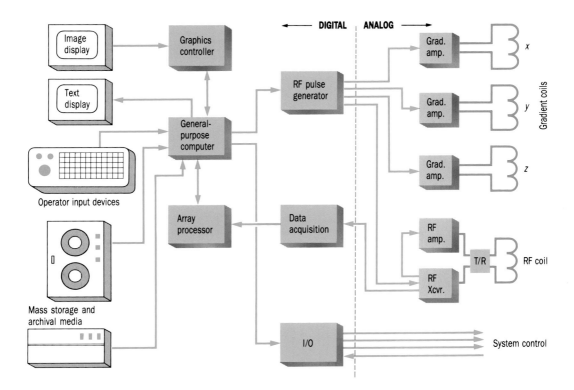

DIGITAL ← | → **ANALOG**

is identical to that of the transmitted exciting radiofrequency (see Figure 1-5). Since the Larmor frequency is determined by the strength of the static magnetic field, it follows that the Larmor frequency will vary in a predictable manner within tissue placed in an inhomogeneous magnetic field. That inhomogeneity results when a gradient coil is turned on at the same time as the RF coil that emits the Larmor frequency. This can be used to create the selective excitation of tissue within a single slice.

Useful clinical information depends on receiving, analyzing, and displaying the analog radiofrequency signals from the excited protons. This requires collecting the data so that they can be spatially encoded and transferred into a digital domain for further processing (Figure 1-6). There are

Figure 1-6 *MRI scanning device. A general-purpose computer operating in a digital domain is used to control various operations in the analog domain, including the magnetic gradient coils and the RF antenna for its transmission (T) and receiver (R) functions. After the RF signal is received, it is converted from analog to digital for processing within the computer and displayed on the image display graphic device as well as the printing device. Other digital and analog interfaces are provided by the input/output (I/O) systems.*

Redrawn with permission from Atlas SW: Magnetic Resonance Imaging of the Brain and Spine. *New York: Raven Press; 1991.*

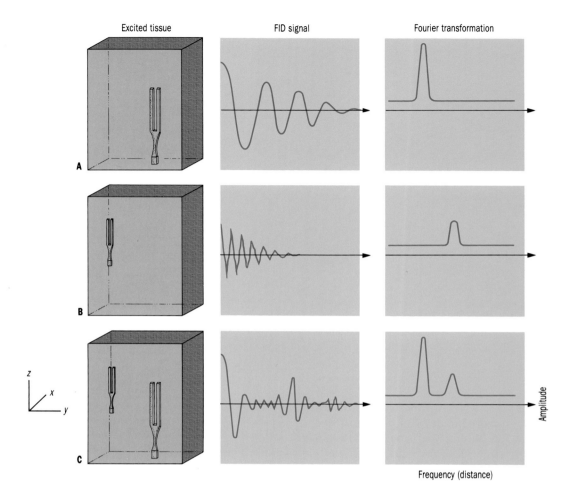

Excited tissue | FID signal | Fourier transformation

Amplitude

Frequency (distance)

Figure 1-7 *Extraction of spatial information, (A,B) Fourier transformation. (C) The sounds emitted by two tuning forks originating from the same volume merge to produce a complex wave form. Fourier transformation (right) identifies the source and amplitude of the two signals. RF signals emitted from relaxing protons at slightly different positions within a signal slice of tissue undergoing MRI scanning emit signals that are measured as free induction decay (FID). The protons at slightly different distances along the y axis emit slightly different resonant frequencies, indicated by large and small tuning forks. Frequency-encoding analysis is performed while the magnetic field gradient is switched on.*

two methods in general clinical use for spatially encoding MRI data: frequency encoding and phase encoding. Frequency encoding uses an antenna to record the FID frequency spectrum produced while the magnetic field gradient is switched on. The protons excited at different positions within the plane will resonate at different frequencies based on their position in the plane (Figure 1-7). The combined signal from such protons can be subjected to Fourier analysis, and projection of their relative location and intensity can be made. Thousands of repeated determinations at many angles within the plane can be made as the gradient is rotated. The gradient coil is not physically rotated, but is arranged to produce the same result as the "slip ring" on a CT scanner, which does physically rotate to send and receive data.

Phase encoding of spatial information takes advantage of the fact that the excitation of the protons and their subsequent relaxation take place at slightly different times, as a function of location within the magnetic field. Thus, phase encoding measures the distance-related delay of the return of the FID signal after the magnetic field gradient is turned off. The gradient coil is turned on after the RF pulse but before the antenna records data. Thousands of repeated determinations are obtained at different gradient strengths on each repetition. The gradient-coil strength can be altered by varying the current strength and direction in the coil.

Spatial encoding is thus based on only one physical principle, whether the technique used is frequency encoding or phase encoding: both measure the FID signal emitted. The only difference is that the frequency-encoding gradient is detected while the magnetic gradient is on, whereas the phase-encoding gradient is recorded after the gradient is turned off. The signal intensity, represented on a two-dimensional projection as a *pixel* (picture element), is proportional to the number of protons precessing within a three-dimensional *voxel* (volume element) within the acquisition matrix. Repeated measurements at all projections in the transverse (x,y) plane are used to calculate the signal intensity at each pixel within the plane. The digital methods of calculation and image construction are similar to those used in computed tomography.

1-1-3 T1 and T2 Defined

Except for magnet strength, the various parameters by which MRI techniques and images are characterized are mostly related to time. T1 and T2 are time constants resulting from inherent tissue characteristics that correspond to the behavior of protons whose nuclei precess in response to applied magnetic and radiofrequency stimuli (Table 1-1). TR (repetition time), TE (echo time), and TI (interpulse time) are time intervals selected by the personnel performing the scan and are independent of any inherent tissue characteristics; these time intervals are discussed in Section 1-1-4.

TABLE 1-1

T1 and T2 in Various Mammalian Tissues at 1.5 T

Tissue	T1 (msec)	T2 (msec)
Muscle		
Skeletal	870	47
Heart	870	57
Liver	490	43
Spleen	560	58
Adipose	260	84
Brain		
Gray matter	920	101
White matter	790	92

Reprinted with permission from Bottomley PA, Foster TH, Argersinger RE, et al: A review of normal tissue hydrogen NMR relaxation times and relaxation mechanisms from 1–100 MHz: dependence on tissue type, NMR frequency, temperature, species, excision, and age. Med Physics 1984;11: 425–448.

In MRI scanning, RF pulses of a selected energy and duration are applied to displace the net magnetic vector from the z axis that was imposed by the static magnetic field. In most cases, the selected pulse will change the net magnetic vector by 90° or 180°. The strength required of the pulse is directly related to the magnetic field strength. With a field strength of 1.5 T, pulses of approximately 64 MHz will excite protons. These pulses are employed either singly or in combination, producing different pulse sequences. The term *longitudinal plane* is used for the z axis, the vector of the magnetic field prior to the onset of the RF pulse. When a sufficient RF pulse is given, all of the protons shift and become oriented 90° away from the longitudinal plane. After the pulse is terminated, there will be zero magnetization of the protons in the longitudinal axis, after which the protons will slowly realign with the magnetic field. This exponential process is called *longitudinal relaxation*. It asymptotically approaches a maximum value of 100%. By convention, the time required for proton spins comprising 63% of the vector to return to the longitudinal axis is designated *T1*, the longitudinal (or spin-lattice) relaxation time (Figure 1-8). This type of relaxation occurs as the stimulated protons lose their kinetic energy due to the retarding forces of neighboring nuclei. Spin-lattice relaxation is essentially a thermal reaction, with the transfer of energy as heat from the protons to the surrounding molecular environment (lattice).

The term *transverse plane* is used when the net magnetic vector is in the x,y axis, located 90° away from the longitudinal plane. Immediately after the RF pulse is terminated, the magnetic vectors for all protons in this plane are identical. Due to imperfections in the static magnetic field and local variations in the magnetic moments of neighboring protons and unpaired electrons, some protons are exposed to a stronger field than others and precess at a faster rate than adjacent protons. The interaction of the magnetic moments of the faster-precessing with the slower-precessing protons causes loss of energy and entropy. The protons exchange their spins with their neighbors—thus the term *spin-spin relaxation*. In a quantum-mechanical model, parallel and antiparallel protons are converted to the opposite state. This leads to a dephasing of the proton spins and causes a rapid dispersion of the magnetic vector with regard to a three-dimensional frame of reference (Figure 1-9). The magnetic vectors thus spread out like the opening of a fan within the transverse plane from their initial location in one direction along the *y* axis. This process of loss of phase coherence among spins is called *transverse relaxation*. By convention, the transverse (spin-spin) relaxation time, or *T2*, is the time required for 63% of the magnetic field in the transverse plane created by the RF pulse to dissipate. This reflects the time-dependent interaction of proton spins, causing nuclei to precess at different rates and deviate from the uniform motion created on initial excitation.

Longitudinal magnetization increases after the termination of the RF pulse (with a time constant of T1), while transverse magnetization decreases after the termination of the RF pulse (with a time constant of T2). T1 relaxation and T2 re-

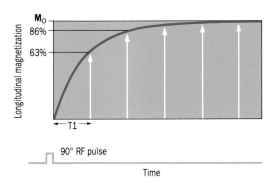

Figure 1-8 *T1 relaxation. T1 is the time required for 63% of the protons comprising the net magnetic vector to return to the longitudinal plane after the cessation of a 90° RF pulse. The 63% is an arbitrary value called the* time constant *for an exponential process.* M_0 *is the maximal value and is not achieved until several multiples of T1 have passed. If the repetition time (TR) is equal to T1, longitudinal remagnetization will not have time to be fully completed.*

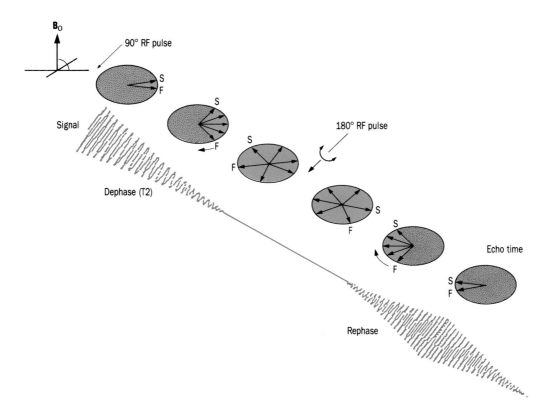

Figure 1-9 *Spin-echo and T2 relaxation. After a 90° RF pulse, the protons are initially all directed along a single axis in the transverse plane and are said to be* in phase. *Thereafter, the faster-precessing and the slower-processing protons interact magnetically and their spins begin to dephase rapidly within the transverse plane so that their vectors spread to occupy an ever-enlarging sector and ultimately a disc. (What is illustrated is a pure T2 effect; the actual process involves a combination of T2 and T1 relaxation so that the* disc illustrated becomes conical, as shown in Figure 1-10.) The application of a 180° refocusing pulse eliminates the effects of static magnetic field inhomogeneities, so that most spins are in phase at the first-echo time. Some residual dephasing is present at the echo owing to T2 effects, which cannot be reversed by the refocusing pulse. The 180° refocusing pulse can be repeated after the first echo is received (compare Figure 1-15). (F = proton spins with faster precession; S = proton spins with slower precession)* Redrawn with permission from Edelman RR, Hesselink JR: Clinical Magnetic Resonance Imaging. Philadelphia: WB Saunders Co; 1990.*

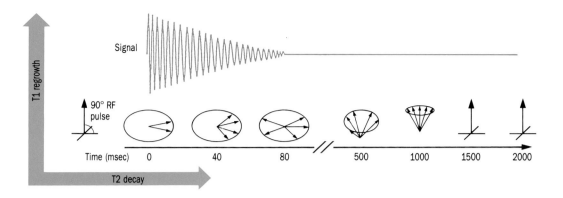

laxation occur simultaneously, but T2 relaxation is completed much more rapidly than T1 relaxation (Figure 1-10). At the end of transverse relaxation, the magnetic vectors can be represented as located along the edge of a disc in the transverse plane. They are then brought into the shape of a cone of decreasing diameter during longitudinal relaxation. The tissue characteristics associated with T1 and T2 are discussed in Section 1-1-5.

1-1-4 TR and TE Defined

An MRI examination protocol is described in part by the RF bursts used in its performance. The operator of the procedure sets the time between pulses, which is called the *repetition time* (TR). This represents the waiting time between cycles of excitation and relaxation. Allowing full longitudinal relaxation to occur (TR > T1) after an RF pulse prolongs the examination time. However, repeating the RF pulse with TR less than the average T1 leads to less signal strength and a more cluttered image (Figure 1-11). These patterns of RF bursts are called *pulse se-*

Figure 1-10 *T1 and T2 relaxation compared. Following a single 90° RF pulse, T1 relaxation and T2 relaxation are simultaneous processes. Note that T2 relaxation is completed much more rapidly than T1 relaxation. The signal emitted represents both T1 and T2 relaxation according to the characteristics of the protons within the tissue. Note that the amplitude of the signal falls rapidly by the time the protons have dephased or are close to the transverse plane during T2 decay.*
Redrawn with permission from Edelman RR, Hesselink JR: Clinical Magnetic Resonance Imaging. *Philadelphia: WB Saunders Co; 1990.*

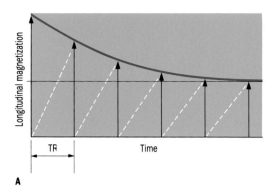

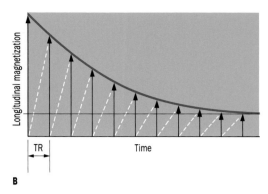

Figure 1-11 *Equilibrium magnetization and magnetic saturation. (A) Greater equilibrium longitudinal magnetization results with a long TR between series of several RF pulses. (B) With a short TR, the equilibrium magnetization is less and the saturation of the protons is greater. In a series of repeated 90° pulses, a short TR is shown to decrease the residual or equilibrium amount of longitudinal magnetization, as compared to a long TR. Decreased equilibrium magnetization is associated with decreased signal strength on T1-weighted images. When 90° RF pulses are repeated with sufficiently rapid succession, the protons realign along the longitudinal meridian but without a net magnetic vector. When the protons align with equal numbers in the parallel and antiparallel directions, they are said to be* saturated; *this phenomenon forms the basis for saturation-recovery scanning. The solid lines represent the longitudinal relaxation following each pulse. The top curve (in color) connects the maximum relaxation at the end of each repetition.*

quences. Typical examples of pulse sequences used in MRI scanning are SR (saturation recovery), SE (spin echo), and IR (inversion recovery).

The effect of varying only TR affects the appearance of tissues. A series of 90° RF pulses followed by the immediate acquisition of the FID signal is shown in Figure 1-12. The illustration presumes that TR is much longer than T1, resulting in an equal FID amplitude after each pulse and thus indicating that complete relaxation occurred prior to the next RF pulse. The signal intensity that is related to T1 relaxation time is illustrated in Figure 1-13, which has been calculated from data similar to those in Table 1-2. Note that the results can be considered in three regions: When TR < 2 sec, the relative signal intensities are white matter (WM) > gray matter (GM) and >> cerebrospinal fluid (CSF); when TR > 2 sec and < 5 sec, GM > WM > CSF; and when TR > 5 sec, CSF > GM > WM. The first pattern is T1-weighted and the last is described as proton-density-weighted.

SR (saturation recovery) sequences record the RF signal emitted by the protons after a series of 90° pulses with interpulse intervals approximately less than or equal to an average tissue T1, 0.1 to 1.5 sec

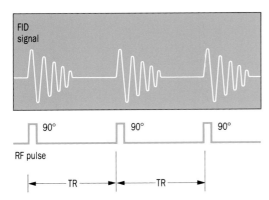

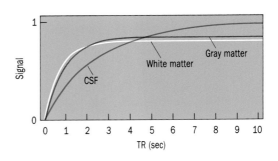

Figure 1-12 *Signal produced by a train of RF pulses separated by a repetition time of TR. The free induction decay (FID) signal is measured immediately after each pulse.*

Figure 1-13 *MRI signal calculated as a function of the pulse repetition time TR for gray matter (GM), white matter (WM), and cerebrospinal fluid (CSF), using the parameters of Table 1-2 and assuming typical relaxation times in proton densities. It is assumed that 90° pulses are applied every TR sec and the signal is collected immediately thereafter. At short TR (TR < 2 sec), the relative signal intensities are WM > GM >> CSF and the resultant image is said to be T1-weighted. At longer TR (TR > 2 sec and < 5 sec), the relative signal intensities are GM > WM > CSF. Finally, at TR > 5 sec, the relative signal intensities are CSF > GM > WM and the resultant images are said to be proton-density-weighted. Gray matter and white matter are isointense when TR is approximately 2 sec and also below 0.5 sec. Note that CSF is essentially isointense with gray and white matter when TR is in the vicinity of 5 sec. If TR is allowed to become greater than 5 sec, CSF will have the highest signal intensity while the proton density of the gray and white matter will provide contrast for the brain. In this illustration, TE is held constant at 15 msec, causing CSF to have lower signal intensity than brain when TR < 5 sec. In clinical T2-weighted imaging, CSF has a higher signal than brain at TR > 2 sec because TE > 30 msec on second-echo images. Compare Figure 1-20.*

Redrawn with permission from Atlas SW: Magnetic Resonance Imaging of the Brain and Spine. *New York: Raven Press; 1991.*

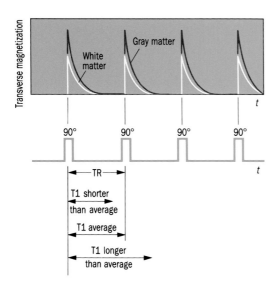

Figure 1-14 *Saturation-recovery pulse sequence. A series of 90° RF pulses is given, separated by TR that is equal to average tissue T1. Relaxation is not complete between pulses. The tissue represented by the curve printed in white has a shorter T1 relaxation time than the tissue characterized by the curve printed in gray. Gray matter has a shorter T1 relaxation time than white matter. Since the FID signal will be related to the transverse magnetization, contrast on the printed image will result because the gray matter will produce a greater signal intensity than white matter for tissues of equal proton density.*

(Figure 1-14). *Saturation* is defined in magnetic resonance as an equilibrium condition in which an equal number of protons are aligned with and against a magnetic field and no further absorption of the RF pulse will take place. Thus, the vector sum is zero and there is no net magnetic vector. Saturation can be produced by repeated pulses having interpulse intervals less than T1. The effect of decreasing TR on the equilibrium magnetization series of pulses is shown in Figure 1-11. Repeating TR more frequently than shown will lead to saturation. Relaxation after the final pulse of such a series occurs from an initial condition of no net magnetization, rather than from an initial condition of partial magnetization as would occur after a single RF pulse. Although they take more imaging time, saturation-recovery techniques are used in T1-weighted scans of the sella to remove the effects of unsaturated protons in blood moving through the imaging volume. Saturation-recovery techniques also are useful in removing swallowing and respiratory motion artifacts.

SE (spin echo) sequences are similar to SR sequences, with the addition of 180° pulses between the 90° pulses. SE techniques include an initial 90° pulse followed by two 180° pulses at equal intervals in succession, which generate first and second echoes (or regenerations). The 180° pulse is given in the transverse plane, flipping the magnetic moment of the protons that have already been excited by the RF pulse while keeping them within the same plane. The resulting signal is sampled at a time TE (echo time) after the RF pulse, which is set by the operator to twice the interval between any two consecutive pulses (see Figure 1-9).

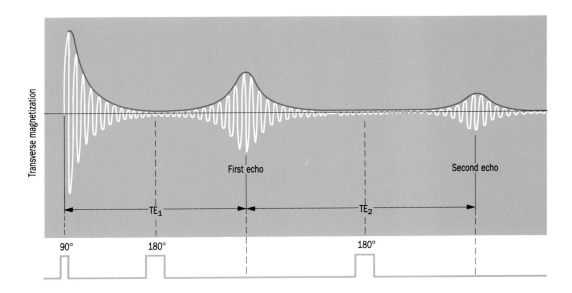

The spin-echo technique minimizes the effects of inhomogeneities in the static magnetic field. The cycle can be thought of as flipping the protons into phase at the end of the pulse. The protons rapidly dephase due to the T2 relaxation but are brought back into phase (rephased) by the 180° RF pulse. The resultant signal is measured again. The first-echo signal is weighted between T1 and T2, while the second-echo signal is T2-weighted. Because a T2 (second echo) image may be required, the first-echo signal can be obtained with no extra scan time, although there is additional cost associated with computing and printing the first-echo images. Depending on the parameters used for scanning, the first-echo images are often called *proton-density-weighted images.*

The first spin echo is received before application of the RF pulse that causes the second echo (Figure 1-15). The TE times will be shown on the scan; thus, the first-echo scan might be TE 30 (the indi-

Figure 1-15 *Use of a spin-echo technique to produce a T2-weighted signal due to signal decay (T2 contrast). The pulse sequence is a 90° RF pulse at the onset followed by two 180° RF refocusing pulses. The first 180° pulse is given at 1/2 the time at which the first echo will be recorded, and the second 180° pulse is given after the recording of the first signal and at 1/2 the time from the initial pulse to the time when the second echo will be recorded. The first and second echoes, TE_1 and TE_2, are asymmetric in this example.*

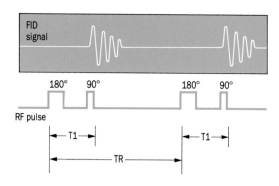

FID signal

180°   90°   180°   90°

RF pulse

←— T1 —→   ←— T1 —→

←————— TR —————→

Figure 1-16 *Inversion-recovery pulse sequence. The initial RF pulse is sufficient to provide a 180° inversion of the net magnetic vector of the protons and bring them into the nonequilibrium condition of antiparallel orientation. TI is the time interval between the inversion and the application of a 90° RF pulse. During TI, the proton spins relax partially, some of them returning to the parallel orientation. Because protons oriented in the longitudinal direction cannot be detected, they are flipped into the transverse plane by the application of the 90° pulse, where they produce a measurable signal.*

cation 1/2 is optional but serves to show it is a first echo). The TE for the second echo may be TE 80 (2/2 indicates that this is a second-echo scan). The 180° RF pulses are given at 1/2 TE so that, for the cycle just described, the 180° RF pulses occur at 15 (30/2) and 70 (30 + 80/2) msec after the initial 90° RF pulse. This pulse sequence is called *asymmetric* because of the unequal TE for the first and second echoes. Asymmetric echo times are often used for examining the orbit because a short first TE will be proton-density-weighted and may increase contrast between the optic nerve and cerebrospinal fluid. The brain is often examined with asymmetric echo times, but other examiners prefer longer first-echo times with resultant identical first and second times (eg, 45 msec). Such symmetric echo times remove the constant-velocity component of the artifacts produced by moving blood. The longer T1 time of a symmetric spin-echo study of the brain may serve to differentiate on the first echo a periventricular plaque in multiple sclerosis from the adjacent cerebrospinal fluid, which could wash out the plaque on the second echo. Variations in TR also affect the contrast. When TR is of the order of 2 sec, the CSF would be hypointense on the first echo; however, when TR > 4 sec, the CSF will be hyperintense at all echo times (see Figure 1-13).

IR (inversion recovery) sequences use initial 180° pulses in the longitudinal plane followed by a 90° pulse and immediate acquisition of the FID signal (Figure 1-16). The interpulse time is designated *TI* (not to be confused with the alphanumeric designation *T1*). Partial recovery of the longitudinal relaxation as a function of TR is measured in the transverse plane by the application of the 90° RF pulse. In

MRI examinations of the orbits, IR is often used with a short TI; this is designated a *STIR* (Short Tau Inversion Recovery) image. At an optimum TI (about 0.4 sec in Figure 1-17), white matter has very little signal. One of many fat-suppression techniques useful in imaging the orbit, STIR is especially valuable when combined with contrast agents, so that a contrast-enhanced tumor will produce an intense signal while normal orbital fat does not on a T1-weighted image.

Alteration of the TR/TE ratio (length of time between 90° pulses/length of time between 180° pulses) determines the signal intensity of the MRI scan, creating T1-weighted, T2-weighted, and proton-density-weighted images. At the time of writing, a new generation of pulse sequences and imaging techniques is coming into clinical use. These are described by a number of terms, including fast imaging, fast low-angle shot (FLASH), ultrafast imaging, reduced-pulse flip angle, gradient-echo pulse sequences, and gradient-echo pulse sequences with conservation of the steady state (GRASS), among others. These techniques hold promise for improved definition of the optic nerve, cerebral hemorrhage, and arteriovenous malformations and for a general reduction of imaging time and cost.

1-1-5 T1 and T2 Relaxation

Protons (hydrogen ions) are present in tissues as a consequence of the presence of water at tissue pH. Even without flow produced by external forces, free water molecules surrounding a hydrogen ion move rapidly and their rotational and translational Brownian movement produces rapid fluctuation in the magnetic fields adjacent to the protons. T2 relaxa-

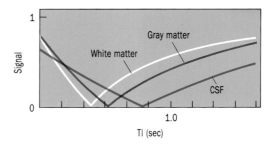

Figure 1-17 *MRI signal calculated as a function of the inversion time TI, assuming a pulse TR of 2.5 sec and the parameters of Table 1-2 for gray matter, white matter, and CSF. It is assumed that 90° pulses are applied every 2.5 sec and the signal is collected immediately after each pulse. Note the multiple crossover points at which gray matter, white matter, and CSF are predicted to be isointense. Furthermore, the inflection points at signal = 0 correspond to TI values, at which time the signal is nulled because the net magnetic vector is in the x,y plane halfway relaxed between the antiparallel and the parallel orientation. This occurs when TI = 0.69 T1 of the tissue.*

Redrawn with permission from Atlas SW: Magnetic Resonance Imaging of the Brain and Spine. *New York: Raven Press; 1991.*

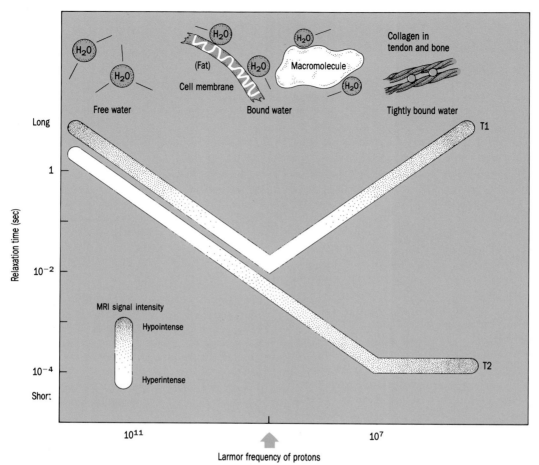

Figure 1-18 *Relaxation time of protons versus frequency (Hz) of molecular motion of water molecules. Free water has rapid diffusion and long T1 and T2 times (free-water region). Bound water associated with restricted motion has shorter T1 and T2 times (bound-water region). Note that the T1 relaxation time of bound water is efficiently shortened as a function of its frequency of molecular motion. The clinical differentiation of biological fluids (CSF and vitreous) from tissues occurs in the region represented by the right half of the bound-water region. Here T1 becomes much longer than T2. High signal intensity is represented by the light regions of the T1 and T2 curves. On T1-weighted images, high signal intensity is associated with short T1 times so that fatty tissue will be characteristically bright. On T2-weighted images, the high signal intensity is associated with long T2 times so that free water and edema in tissue will be characteristically bright. Note that free water molecules diffuse randomly in all directions. Bound water is associated with macromolecules and cell membranes and has T1 and T2 relaxation times that are shorter than those of free water. Collagen has tightly bound water with long T1 relaxation times and very short T2 relaxation times.*

Redrawn and modified with permission from Edelman RR, Hesselink JR: Clinical Magnetic Resonance Imaging. *Philadelphia: WB Saunders Co; 1990.*

tion times are generally faster than T1 relaxation times. These molecular water–proton interactions accelerate T1 and T2 relaxation. Water molecules attached (bound) to proteins or to cell membranes (this is especially prominent in fat cells) move less rapidly than unattached (free) water molecules within tissue (Figure 1-18). Water molecules in moving blood move rapidly. In adipose tissue and proteinaceous solutions, limited movement of water molecules occurs at a fluctuation rate equal to that of the resonant frequencies of the protons. Such solutions have rapid T1 and intermediate T2 relaxation times. However, in pure water, the molecules fluctuate more rapidly than the protons and do not affect them as much, giving pure water long T1 and T2 relaxation times, measured in seconds as opposed to milliseconds. When water molecules are very tightly bound to collagen in tendons and scar tissue, their slow fluctuation promotes T2 relaxation but not T1 relaxation. Thus, such tissues have T2 relaxation times of less than 50 msec, while the T1 relaxation times may be in the vicinity of 1 sec. Slower-moving molecules such as proteins produce less rapid fluctuations in the magnetic field experienced by their protons and do not affect T1 relaxation as much as the faster-moving free water molecules. In biologic tissues, water is often bound to proteins, causing a change in the T1 relaxation of that protein. Efficient shortening of T1 relaxation occurs in the region of the curve representing the movement of water molecules bound to proteins and cell membranes, which restricts molecular motion compared to free water molecules. Perturbations in the bound-water and free-water content of tissues contribute to the contrast of abnormal from normal tissues.

1-1-6 Factors Determining the Appearance of MRI Scans

Image appearance of normal tissues on MRI depends on four major characteristics:

1. The proton density of structures contributes the majority of information concerning the structures. Tissues with higher proton density produce the most intense signals.

2. The time between the RF pulse and the sampling is represented in the parameters TR and TE and controls the T1 and T2 weighting of the images (Figure 1-19).

3. Flow is an important consideration in fluids that do not remain stationary. If protons are stimulated by the RF pulse and leave the slice being scanned before the image is sampled, then no signal will be seen. Similarly, the protons that have come into the slice after the RF pulse have not been exposed to the pulse, and such protons will not contribute to the image. As a result, a flow void is seen where rapid flow exists. Thus, large vessels appear dark on both T1- and T2-weighted images unless special techniques are used to display them (ie, MR angiography).

4. The electron clouds around atomic nuclei shield them from the applied magnetic field during the RF pulse, creating alterations in the local field that the nuclei encounter. For example, protons associated with water have a different Larmor frequency than protons associated with lipids or proteins because of differences in the electron cloud configuration.

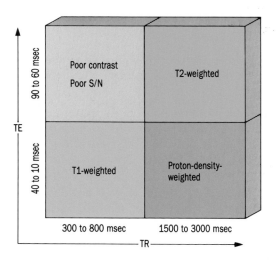

Figure 1-19 *Image contrast as a function of TR and TE. The 40 to 10 msec time shown in the bottom half corresponds to the first-echo times used clinically, while the upper half corresponds to the second-echo times. The TR shown on the right half corresponds to the TR used in a spin-echo technique, thus producing a proton-density-weighted scan on the first echo and a T2-weighted scan on the second echo. The T1-weighted signal is produced when TR is in the range shown on the right half. (S/N = signal-to-noise ratio)*
Redrawn with permission from Edelman RR, Hesselink JR: Clinical Magnetic Resonance Imaging. *Philadelphia: WB Saunders Co; 1990.*

The difference in resonant frequency between the applied and the locally perceived fields creates a so-called *chemical shift*, which is responsible for phase-contrast effects between fat and water (see Figure 5-1). This occurs when the computer program analyzes the shift in frequency as a shift in distance, because that is how the gradient coil is used to determine position in a plane. A shift in frequency is the cue to the computer that there has been a shift in distance proportional to the change in frequency. This chemical shift artifact can produce black-and-white shadows on opposite sides of the optic nerve, simulating a tumor.

Table 1-2 provides characteristics useful in differentiating the different types of MRI protocols. Note that gray matter and white matter have essentially equal proton densities, thus limiting the usefulness of this technique for differentiating normal anatomy. Look at the vitreous cavity and the cerebrospinal fluid to make an initial evaluation of the weighting of a scan. If normal vitreous and cerebrospinal fluid are black, the scan is T1-weighted; if they are white, the scan is T2-weighted. If they are gray, the image is likely to be a first-echo or proton-density-weighted scan.

There is insufficient appreciation of the ability of MRI to adequately image bone and detect fractures. It is true that water molecules in cortical bone are tightly bound and few in number, producing no detectable signal. The black image of cortical bone can be appreciated as having contrast with regard to adjacent medullary bone, muscle, and fat. Moreover, hyperintense signals due to the intrusion of hemorrhage and edema into the normal low signal of cortical bone should alert to the presence of a fracture or tumor.

MEDICAL COLLEGE OF PENNSYLVANIA
AND HAHNEMANN UNIVERSITY
UNIVERSITY LIBRARY, CENTER CITY

TABLE 1-2

Factors Affecting MRI Signal Intensity

Protocol	Imaging Parameters			Relative Intensity of Signal					
	TI	TR	TE	Bone/Air	Fat	Vitreous/ CSF	Nerve/ Muscle	Gray matter	White matter
T1-weighted	None	600	15	0	+ +	− −	+	−	+
T2-weighted	None	2500	90	0	− −	+ + +	−	+	±
STIR	150	1500	20	0	− −	+ +	+ +	+ +	−
Proton density (%)					9.6	10.8	9.7	10.6	10.6

Top: Typical imaging parameters used in clinical magnetic resonance images of the orbit. Typical signal intensities for various tissues are compared. + indicates brighter than average intensity; − indicates less than average intensity. Bottom: The proton densities of various tissues are shown and expressed as a percentage of MRI-visible protons in tissue as compared to pure water. Note that the differences between tissues are small. This limits the usefulness of proton-density-weighted images.

1-1-7 T1-weighted Images

T1-weighted images (Figures 4-1 ... 4-13) are created by imaging with short TR values (200 to 1000 msec) and short TE values (15 to 25 msec). Because it is impractical to use a TE of 0, all T1-weighted images have some degree of T2 weighting, which increases with a longer TE. Tissues that inherently have a shorter T1 will have greater signal intensity at a given TR than those with a longer T1 (Figure 1-20). Fat has a short T1, while gray matter, white matter, muscle, and cerebrospinal fluid demonstrate increasingly long T1 relaxation times. T1-weighted images provide better anatomic detail than T2-weighted images because the shorter time required to obtain images means less artifact induced by movement, including vascular pulsations of the brain.

T1 weighting is particularly good for imaging detail in the orbit (Figures 2-1 ... 2-25). Excellent contrast is observed between the high signal intensity of fat and the less intense signals of muscle and vessels. T1-weighted MRI can be useful for evaluating choroidal melanoma because of

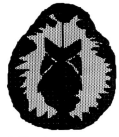

A TR = 1 sec   **B** TR = 3 sec

Figure 1-20 *Theoretical MRI signal calculated as a function of the pulse repetition time (TR), assuming 90° pulses are applied every TR second and the signal is collected immediately thereafter. (A) T1-weighted (~1 sec). At short TR, the relative signal intensities are WM > GM >> CSF. The gray matter is relatively darker than the white matter because it contains more water. (B) Proton-density-weighted (~3 sec). At longer TR, the relative signal intensities are GM > WM > CSF. Note that GM and WM have reversed signal intensities but that the brain still has a higher signal than CSF. (Compare Figure 1-13, where TR = 1 sec corresponds to part A and TR = 3 corresponds to part B of this figure. Also compare Figure 1-21.)*

Reprinted with permission from Latchaw RE: MR and CT Imaging of the Head, Neck and Spine. *2nd ed. St Louis: Mosby-Yearbook; 1991.*

stable free radicals within melanin having paramagnetic properties that decrease both T1 and T2 relaxation times. This makes the tumor brighter on T1-weighted images and darker on T2-weighted images. Acute and subacute intraocular hemorrhages can also be evaluated. Outside the orbit, high signal intensity on T1-weighted images is normally seen in the cavernous sinus (excluding the internal carotid artery, which is seen as a flow void), posterior pituitary gland, pituitary stalk, sinus mucosa, small veins with slow flow rates, and dural reflections (ie, the falx cerebri and the tentorium cerebelli). The dura on T1-weighted images behaves somewhat like gray matter in signal; the rich amount of vessels (especially slow blood flow veins) gives dura the increased signal. This is especially true of the tentorium cerebelli (on CT it is the higher-attenuating blood in vessels that allows the tentorium cerebelli to be identified).

1-1-8 T2-weighted Images

Increasing TR to greater than 2000 msec and the second TE to more than 70 msec produces an image with T2 weighting (Figures 4-14 ... 4-16). Because TR is set at a value much greater than an average T1, most of the T1 effect is eliminated. However, eliminating T1 characteristics altogether would increase scanning time considerably. As a result, T2-weighted images still possess a minimal amount of T1 characteristics. Tissues with low T2 values lose their signal more rapidly than

those with high T2 values, because T2 is a measure of the dephasing of the proton spins (Figures 1-15 and 1-21). The rapidly dephasing protons in tissues with short T2 times emit a wide range of frequencies that are excluded by the receiver, which is narrowly tuned to the Larmor frequency. As a result, the long T2 tissues have a brighter signal than the short T2 tissues—the opposite of T1. To express it another way, those tissues whose protons slowly dephase have a long T2 and a high intensity signal. Examples include water and cerebrospinal fluid. T2-weighted images are less useful for fine anatomic detail than T1-weighted images because of the increased time required for acquisition. However, because of the hyperintense signal associated with perturbations of free water and bound water in tissues affected by edema, demyelination, and tumor infiltration, T2-weighted images are frequently used to screen the brain for disease, demonstrating these changes more dramatically than T1 weighting (see Figure 1-18).

1-1-9 Proton-Density-weighted Images

Proton density refers to the number of MRI-visible protons in a unit volume of tissue. This number increases directly in proportion to water content. The proton density of different tissues differs by at most a few percentage points, producing an image with only modest tissue contrast (Figure 5-1, Table 1-2). Proton-density-weighted images are produced by combining a long TR (greater than 2000 msec) with a short TE (20 to 25 msec). The TR in these images is long enough that essentially all protons have relaxed, minimizing T1 characteristics, and the TE is short

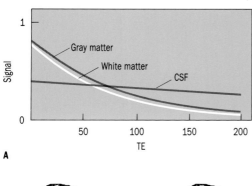

A

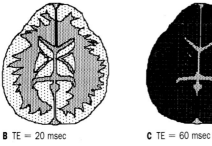

B TE = 20 msec   **C** TE = 60 msec

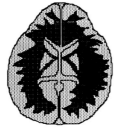

D TE = 100 msec

Figure 1-21 *The signal intensity on T2-weighted scans is a function of echo time for the spin-echo pulse sequence. (A) Theoretical brain signal versus echo time (msec, TE) calculated on the basis of TR = 2 sec. The high signal intensity results from the narrow frequency spectrum emitted by the protons precessing in phase that result in a long T2 signal. The rapidly dephasing protons in tissues with short T2 times emit a wide range of frequencies that are excluded by the receiver, which is narrowly tuned to the Larmor frequency. Note that the cerebrospinal fluid (CSF) will be relatively bright at longer echo times only because fat, gray matter, white matter, muscle, and tightly bound water in tissue all dephase even more quickly. At shorter echo times, CSF has a lower signal intensity due to its long T1. However, as TE increases, the CSF signal intensity eventually surpasses that of GM and WM due to its very long T2 (approximately 1500 msec vs 80 and 70 msec for GM and WM, respectively). The brain contrast shown in B, C, and D correspond to TEs of approximately 20 msec (GM > WM >> CSF), 60 msec (GM = CSF > WM), and 100 msec (CSF > GM > WM). This last image is said to be T2-weighted.*

Reprinted with permission from Latchaw RE: MR and CT Imaging of the Head, Neck and Spine. *2nd ed. St Louis: Mosby-Yearbook; 1991.*

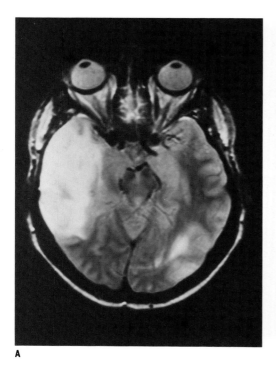

A

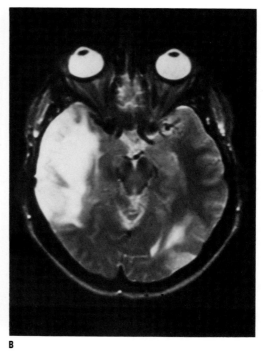

B

Figure 1-22 *Comparison of a proton-density-weighted image with other imaging parameters. These are four axial sections, the first three taken at identical levels through the globe and brain, the latter containing a right frontotemporal lobe oligodendroglioma. (A) Proton-density-weighted image slightly T2-weighted (because TE > 25), showing excellent anatomic detail (note the compression of the cerebral peduncle by the uncus at the tentorial notch and the differentiation of gray and white matter in the occipital lobes). TR = 2500, TE = 30, TA (acquisition time) = 6:04 (minutes:seconds). (B) T2-weighted image showing somewhat less anatomic detail but better definition of the intense signal produced by the free water in the tumor edema and by the CSF in the interpeduncular cistern and the tip of the left occipital horn of the lateral ventricle. TR = 2500, TE = 90, TA = 6:04.*

enough that T2 relaxation is minimized. As a result, a high signal signifies a high proton density in a structure, regardless of its T1 or T2 traits. Although proton-density-weighted images have a characteristically low signal intensity, they are useful for delineating anatomic details in comparison with the high signal intensities seen on T1- and T2-weighted scans, which may be degraded by artifact. In practice, proton-density-weighted and T2-weighted images are obtained during the same SE sequence (Figure 1-22). The initial 90° pulse is given, followed by two consecutive 180° pulses, producing first- and second-echo images (proton-density-weighted and T2-weighted images). Bone and calcified structures produce no signals because the protons are not free to spin, as they are in a freer matrix such as water. Tumors and other pathologic conditions may

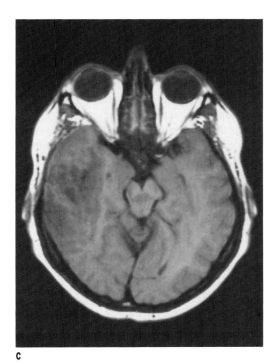

C

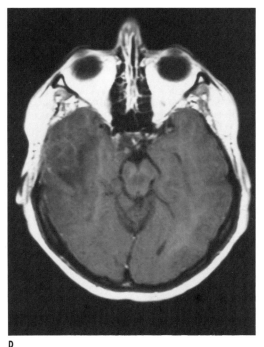

D

have increased proton density, causing decreased contrast on T1-weighted images and increased signal on proton-density-weighted and T2-weighted images.

1-1-10 MRI of Hemorrhage, Blood, and Cerebrospinal Fluid

MRI offers opportunities to image blood, whether intravascular or extravascular, and to detect the movement of blood and cerebrospinal fluid. In some circumstances, this is the desired result; in other circumstances, it leads to undesirable artifacts or loss of information. In each case, a detailed discussion of the MRI appearance is beyond the scope of this monograph. However, certain concepts are necessary for a basic understanding of these subjects.

Magnetic susceptibility is the tendency of a substance to become magnetized or to

Figure 1-22 *(C) T1-weighted image showing that the anatomic detail is distorted by the tumor but on this T1-weighted image the absence of intense signal from the free water could cause the tumor to be overlooked. Note that the vitreous is dark and that the horizontal recti are better defined here than on any of the other images in this series. TR = 600, TE = 15, TA = 1:58. (D) Contrast-enhanced T1-weighted image. The tumor shows minimal enhancement so that the T2-weighted image proves to be the most diagnostic. The horizontal recti are enhanced due to their blood supply and are less contrasted from the orbital fat than they were before. The apparent size of the globes is reduced due to imperfect repositioning in the scanner after injection of the contrast. TR = 600, TE = 15, TA = 1:58. If fat-suppression techniques were used, the brain would look about the same but the orbital fat would be much less intense, improving the visualization of contrast-enhanced structures.*

distort a magnetic field (Figure 1-23). Diamagnetism is a property characteristic of most substances that causes them to weakly repel or decrease an applied magnetic field. A diamagnetic substance has a negative magnetic susceptibility. Conversely, a paramagnetic substance has a positive magnetic susceptibility; it increases the local magnetic field. Paramagnetic substances usually have unpaired electrons and include ferric iron, methemoglobin, molecular oxygen, free radicals, and gadolinium-DTPA (diethylenetriaminepentaacetic acid, an MRI contrast agent). Superparamagnetic materials, such as iron oxides, have large positive magnetic susceptibilities such that they can become transiently magnetized in a magnetic field. Ferromagnetic materials have the largest positive magnetic susceptibility. They become magnetized within a magnetic field and can permanently maintain their magnetization following removal from the magnetic field. Gadolinium-DTPA shortens the relaxation time of protons in the adjacent tissue (relaxivity) and increases the T2 signal (see Section 1-1-11). Tissues with paramagnetic properties have shortened T1 and T2 relaxation times in MRI, because the magnetic properties contribute to the rapid dephasing of the protons and the loss of energy to the lattice. The lattice denotes the organized network of molecules or atoms in crystalline solids and, by extension, in other solids. Such tissues are thus associated with a hyperintense signal on T1-weighted images and a hypointense signal on T2-weighted images. The reader is cautioned that tables comparing the MRI scan intensities of paramagnetic tissues (blood and melanomas, for example) usually compare the tissues to normal gray matter, not to vitreous or cerebrospinal fluid.

Certain types of mascara and tattooed eyeliner employ iron-containing particles that create artifacts. Not only will their location be hyperintense on T1-weighted images and hypointense on T2-weighted images, but they can perturb the local magnetic field and interfere with image reconstruction.

After blood is extravasated and iron escapes from hemoglobin, tissue damage results due to free-radical formation promoted by unchelated iron. The iron atom normally has 6 electrons in its third (d) shell and 2 in its fourth shell (see Figure 1-23). In the ferrous ion (Fe^{++}), all 6 electrons in the d orbital have the same energy. However, in the presence of different ligands, the electrons rearrange in their orbits and exhibit dipoles. Thus, the ferrous ion becomes diamagnetic when attached to oxyhemoglobin and paramagnetic when attached to deoxyhemoglobin. The loss of oxygen from hemoglobin forces a redistribution of the 6 electrons so that 4 unpaired electrons of parallel spin are left over. Because of the unpaired electrons, deoxyhemoglobin is a paramagnetic substance. Intravascular blood has a high content of oxyhemoglobin in arteries and deoxyhemoglobin in veins (Table 1-3). Extravascular blood rapidly loses its oxygen so that the signal produced will be that of deoxyhemoglobin, which has poor magnetic relaxivity because water molecules cannot approach the iron chelated in the porphyrin ring. The conversion of deoxyhemoglobin into methemoglobin changes the configuration so that the iron

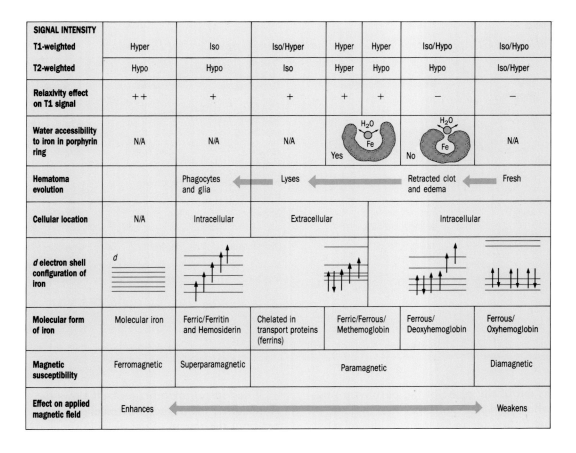

SIGNAL INTENSITY							
T1-weighted	Hyper	Iso	Iso/Hyper	Hyper	Hyper	Iso/Hypo	Iso/Hypo
T2-weighted	Hypo	Hypo	Iso	Hyper	Hypo	Hypo	Iso/Hyper
Relaxivity effect on T1 signal	++	+	+	+	+	−	−
Water accessibility to iron in porphyrin ring	N/A	N/A	N/A	H_2O / Fe — Yes		H_2O / Fe — No	N/A
Hematoma evolution		Phagocytes and glia ←	Lyses ←			Retracted clot and edema ←	Fresh
Cellular location	N/A	Intracellular	Extracellular		Intracellular		
d electron shell configuration of iron	d						
Molecular form of iron	Molecular iron	Ferric/Ferritin and Hemosiderin	Chelated in transport proteins (ferrins)	Ferric/Ferrous/Methemoglobin		Ferrous/Deoxyhemoglobin	Ferrous/Oxyhemoglobin
Magnetic susceptibility	Ferromagnetic	Superparamagnetic	Paramagnetic				Diamagnetic
Effect on applied field	Enhances ←						→ Weakens

Figure 1-23 *Factors affecting the MRI appearance of an intracerebral hemorrhage over time. The diagram shows the configuration of the third electron shell orbitals of iron in relation to the ionic state and biochemical combinations. The relative height of the orbitals reflects increasing energy content. In the presence of ligands, the energy level of the orbitals is increased and they become less equal. The presence of unpaired electron spins (up and down arrows) gives rise to paramagnetic and superparamagnetic states. Both deoxyhemoglobin and methemoglobin are paramagnetic, but their breakdown product, hemosiderin, is superparamagnetic. Water molecules are excluded from deoxyhemoglobin but not from methemoglobin due to their configuration in the porphyrin ring. Entrance of the water shortens T1 relaxation (hyperintense signal) and T2 relaxation (hypointense signal). As long as the met-hemoglobin is aggregated in intact red blood cells, its magnetic-susceptibility properties will contribute to shortening the T2 relaxation. This effect on T2 is lost when lysis of the red cells occurs, with a resultant lengthening of T2, and produces the hyperintensity seen on T2-weighted images of chronic hematomas. A curious phenomenon explains the hypointensity of an acute hematoma seen on a T1-weighted image. The acute blood rapidly deoxygenates and become deoxyhemoglobin, which has a very short T2. Because every T1-weighted image is produced by a process that includes a short TR but an even shorter TE, the TE effect dominates as the absence of relaxivity precludes shortening of T1. Thus, a T2 effect dominates a "T1-weighted image." (N/A = not applicable)*

TABLE 1-3

MRI and CT Appearance in the Center of an Intraparenchymal Cerebral Hemorrhage

Time (Variable)	Biochemical/Cellular Basis	MRI Intensity		CT Density
		T1-weighted	T2-weighted	
Active	Intracellular Fe^{++} oxyhemoglobin	Isodense/ Hypodense	Isodense/ Hypodense	Bright/ Isodense
Hyperacute	Intracellular Fe^{++} oxyhemoglobin	Isodense/ Hypodense	Hyperdense	Bright
	Deoxyhemoglobin	Isodense/ Hypodense	Hypodense	
Acute	Intracellular Fe^{++} deoxyhemoglobin	Isodense	Hypodense	Bright
Late acute	Intracellular Fe^{++} methemoglobin	Hyperdense	Hypodense	Bright/ Isodense
Subacute	Extracellular Fe^{+++} methemoglobin after cell lysis	Hyperdense	Hyperdense	Isodense
Chronic	Methemoglobin (center)	Hyperdense	Hyperdense	Dark/ Isodense
	Hemosiderin (periphery)	Isodense	Hypodense	

is out of the plane of the porphyrin ring, allowing water molecules into proximity with the iron and improving the relaxivity. In a later step in the metabolism of extravasated blood, the ferrous ion of methemoglobin is oxidized to the ferric ion. With the loss of 1 electron, the remaining 5 electrons in the third suborbital are unpaired so that the ferric ion is also paramagnetic in methemoglobin. Methemoglobin has better relaxivity than deoxyhemoglobin because water molecules can approach the iron when the structure of the globin porphyrin is irreversibly changed so that it can no longer "protect" the iron from water molecules.

The red cell membrane itself slows the diffusion of diamagnetic extracellular water from the region of paramagnetism associated with the deoxyhemoglobin in the intracellular compartment. Diffusion is of little importance on a T1-weighted image where TR is short, but it limits detection of a fresh hemorrhage on a T2-weighted image where TR is long, because extracellular water diffuses into the cell and experiences different magnetic fields during the long TR. Once the red cell is lysed, the remaining ferrous ions can be oxidized to the ferric ions. Later and in the more peripheral region of the clot, iron-chelating transfer proteins (the ferrins) and iron storage proteins (ferritin and hemosiderin) are produced. These compounds are found within phagocytes, reticuloendothelial cells, and glial cells. They are superparamagnetic and give a very dark (black) signal on T2-weighted images.

Over time, the effect of these processes is the production of complex changes in the balance of T1 and T2 weighting of the posthemorrhagic signal. Table 1-3 shows an approximate progression of that appearance. It follows that special techniques will be required to evaluate an aneurysm of the carotid artery surrounded by a deoxyhemoglobin thrombus, because both the flowing blood and the thrombus could be dark on both T1- and T2-weighted images. The age of blood in the vitreous can also be estimated by application of this information, bearing in mind that any blood in the vitreous cavity will have a greater proton density than the normal vitreous. The exact time course of a hemorrhage varies so that the clinical dating of actual hemorrhage is notoriously inaccurate.

Flowing blood in large vessels produces black images, with certain exceptions that can cause troublesome artifacts. The technical discussion of these artifacts is beyond the scope of this volume, but a few caveats may be helpful. Beware of masses near large arteries that appear in only one pulse sequence. Flow signals can cause ghost artifacts along the phase-encoding axis (see Figure 4-5). Examples of such artifacts include cerebellar masses simulating cryptic arteriovenous malformations produced by pulsatile flow in the transverse sinuses, pseudoaneurysms of the carotid artery extending into the midbrain, pseudothromboses, and pseudoectasias.

Thrombosis of the cerebral veins and dural sinuses can be optimally detected with MRI. A number of techniques using short TE, cardiac gating, and two- and three-dimensional Fourier transforms (2DFT, 3DFT) are used to differentiate flowing blood from stationary tissues, thus providing the basis for magnetic resonance angiography (MRA).

MRA is a rapidly evolving field that consists of new families of pulse sequences. The goal is not only to rival existing intravascular angiographic radiologic techniques in anatomic clarity and to surpass them in safety but to provide an entirely new form of physiologic information based on the velocity of the flowing fluid. It is possible to selectively image vessels displaying certain peak velocities. For example, the normal systolic peak velocity for the internal carotid artery is in the range of 100 ± 12 cm/sec. Major cerebral venous drainage occurs at about 20 cm/sec. Two fundamental approaches are used for MRA. Time-of-flight angiography detects the flow of fully magnetized blood into the imaging plane in which the tissue is partially saturated by repeated magnetizations with TR much shorter than the T1 of stationary tissues. There is a flow-related enhancement of the moving blood compared to the signal derived from the stationary tissue. Another technique, called *phase-contrast angiography*, uses the phase shifts that occur within moving blood after magnetization to distinguish it from stationary tissue.

Detailed discussion of these evolving techniques is beyond the scope of this work, but it is certain that successful application will require close consultation between those who order the tests and those who interpret them. One reason is that the MRA technique is prone to non-vascular artifacts from stationary structures (eg, a clot) that may appear to be vessels containing moving blood. Conversely, areas of moving blood may not produce a signal for reasons of geometry (a loop that reverses the flow direction in the imaging plane) or because of slow velocity (eg, within arteriovenous malformations).

CSF also is subject to pulsatile and nonpulsatile flow, which can produce effects that are occasionally interesting and often misleading. These CSF-induced motion artifacts can degrade image quality and produce false-negative scans by obscuring disease or false-positive scans by simulating disease. Dependent on the cardiac cycle, CSF undergoes an oscillatory flow in which the CSF is caudally displaced from the ventricular system and ejected into the basilar cisterns as well as into the cranial and spinal subarachnoid spaces during systole. During diastole, CSF returns to its original position. As a consequence, CSF is almost always flowing. T1-weighted images are not as subject to CSF motion artifact as T2-weighted images. Ghost images occur especially when the TR (eg, 2400 msec) approaches an integral multiple of the heart rate (eg, 800 msec). CSF flow-related enhancement can simulate masses or bands within the lateral ventricles, blood within the aqueduct of Sylvius, or masses within the pons or basilar cisterns. False negatives can be produced by CSF flow in the third ventricle, obscuring the details of the temporal lobes along with the temporal horns of the lateral ventricles. Flow-compensation techniques are usually included in imaging protocols, partially suppressing these artifacts. Conversely, CSF flow can be detected using the techniques of MR angiography. The brightest CSF signal will emanate from the regions of greatest flow velocity such as the parapontine cisterns and the space around the cervical spinal cord.

1-1-11 Paramagnetic Contrast Agents

Early studies with nuclear magnetic resonance led to the incorrect expectation that contrast media would not be needed nor enhance the information content in a clinical context. The use of paramagnetic agents to shorten the relaxation time of protons was first reported in 1978. Paramagnetic contrast agents are not directly visualized, unlike more conventional contrast-enhancing agents such as fluorescein and iodinated dyes. These agents have at least 1 unpaired electron and have more than 1000 times the magnetic moment of a proton. In their presence, rapid fluctuation of the local magnetic field will be induced. This fluctuation facilitates the transfer of energy from nearby protons to their lattice and hastens their return to the initial state of longitudinal magnetization.

Of all chemical elements, gadolinium possesses the greatest relaxation-shortening property because of its 7 unpaired electrons. It is toxic in vivo in small amounts, binding to calcium channels in muscle and neural tissues, blocking both muscle contraction and neurotransmission. Fortunately, when chelated with DTPA, gadolinium forms a stable compound that does not diminish its paramagnetic properties. The agent is eliminated renally, with greater than 90% excretion in 24 hours. Gadolinium-DTPA does not cross intact plasma membranes or the blood–brain endothelial barrier. Disruption of the endothelium results in intense enhancement due to influx of the agent into the perivascular tissue. In the usual clinical doses, gadolinium has a more marked effect on shortening T1 relaxation times than T2 relaxation times (see Figure 1-18, noting the effect on signal intensity of decreasing relaxation time from 1 to 10^{-2} sec). As a result, studies with gadolinium are usually performed on T1-weighted scans. Changes of 10% to 20% in tissue relaxivity are sufficient for detection with clinical MRI. In the diagnosis of orbital disorders, gadolinium is often combined with a fat-suppression technique to allow enhancing lesions to be separated from adjacent orbital fat with its characteristically intense signal. This technique is particularly useful in the evaluation of meningiomas involving the optic nerve.

When these agents are used according to the directions provided, their record of clinical safety has been excellent. Following administration of gadolinium-DTPA, headache, injection-site coldness, hypotension, hives, asthmatic attacks with bronchospasm (rare), and a transient rise in serum iron have been observed. In patients with hemolytic and sickle cell anemias, gadolinium-DPTA may be contraindicated.

1-1-12 Spatial Resolution

Spatial resolution in MRI is limited by the size of the sampling matrix. The signal intensity, represented on a two-dimensional projection as a *pixel* (picture element), is proportional to the number of protons precessing within a three-dimensional *voxel* (volume element) within the acquisition matrix. Pixel size is determined by the field of view, FOV; the horizontal and vertical distance from one side of the image to the other is expressed in centimeters and is divided by the acquisition matrix, M. (The acquisition matrix is not identical with the interpolated display matrix, which may be 512 × 512 or greater.) With standard parameters of FOV = 25 cm and M = 256 × 256, the pixel size is approximately 1 mm^2. The signal intensity within each of 62,500 voxels will need to be acquired and computed for each slice! Increased resolution is gained at the expense of increased scanning time. In practice, the acquisition pixel size is controlled by selecting the FOV and only secondarily by setting the acquisition matrix. FOV can be decreased by increasing the strength of the frequency-encoding and phase-encoding gradients. Decreasing FOV by 1/2 reduces the pixel area by 1/2 and the voxel volume by a factor of 4. This worsens the signal-to-noise (S/N) ratio because the density of protons within the voxel determines the signal intensity. The noise level within the scanner is produced by random motion of charged molecules and

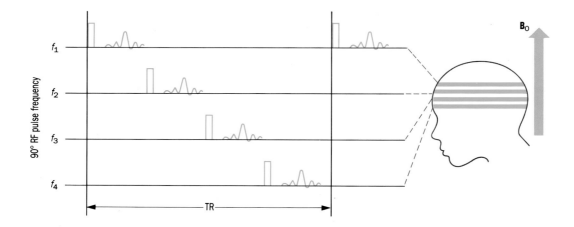

Figure 1-24 *Multiple-slice imaging saves time by allowing sequential imaging of other slices while the first slice is recovering (TR) from its initial 90° pulse. Each of the four slices shown is missed by a pulse at a different frequency (f_1 ... f_4) according to its calculated Larmor frequency within the magnetic gradient (B$_0$). The 90° RF pulse is represented by a rectangular wave, and the resultant free induction decay (FID) signal by the wave form.*

the electrical resistance of the magnetic coil. Because the noise is related only to the magnetic field strength, decreasing FOV geometrically decreases the S/N ratio. Nonetheless, spatial detail can be improved by decreasing FOV even at the expense of a grainier image produced by decreasing S/N. Similarly, decreasing slice thickness decreases the volume within the voxel. This also increases resolution at the expense of decreased S/N.

The total acquisition time is determined by (1) TR, (2) the number of columns in the acquisition matrix, and (3) the number of repetitions (the number of times the scanning is repeated). These numbers are printed on the hard copy of the image as TR, M, and ACQ or NEX. Assuming the acquisition matrix and the number of repetitions to be identical, a T2-weighted image with a TR of 2000 msec will take $3\frac{1}{3}$ times longer to obtain than a T1-weighted image with a TR of 600 msec. To decrease scanning time, either NEX or M must be decreased. It is possible to use an M of 256 × 128 to cut scanning time in half, but doing so will also reduce the resolution in the *y* direction by half and can induce artifacts along the sides of the image. The number of acquisitions may be as low as 2 in voxels with sufficient proton density, but must be increased when the voxel size is small or the signal is weak.

1-1-13 Multiple-Slice Imaging

Clinical scanning is limited by patient movement over time so that it is desirable to increase the speed of data acquisition. Decreasing imaging time is one of the most important goals in equipment design and in imaging-sequence selection. One technique that is used to decrease imaging time is the sequential measurement of multiple parallel slices during the time that the protons in the first slice of the series can recover from their initial RF pulse and before the slice can be re-excited to measure other points on its *y* axis (Figure 1-24). Multiple-slice imaging helps to alleviate the limited repetition rate (TR) required for the initial magnetization to be largely or completely degraded prior to remagnetization for successive images. Typical acquisition protocols involve 5 to 20 slices at a time. One artifact caused by multiple-slice imaging is the disappearance of vessels at the entrance slice that contain protons not yet magnetized in the moving blood.

1-1-14 Surface-Coil Techniques

In neuroimaging, surface coils may be used to evaluate superficial structures, such as the spinal cord, inner ear, and orbit. These coils are applied directly to the region of interest. The whole-body cylindrical coil within the scanner provides the excitation stimulus, and the surface coil is used only for detection. Using the surface coil for receiving the RF signal is common for orbital coils, but in some magnets the head coil may be both sender and receiver of the RF signal. Because the coil covers only a small region, it allows high resolution due to an improved S/N ratio. Within the orbit, surface coils allow excellent resolution back to the apex. However, if a lesion is thought to extend through the optic foramen or the superior orbital fissure, surface coils may not be useful. In addition, surface coils are more sensitive to movement than stationary coils and may increase movement artifact on T2-weighted images. While excellent anatomic and pathophysiologic data concerning orbital structures have been obtained with surface coils, there are few clinical problems for which surface coils are the only relevant solution.

1-1-15 Contraindications

Contraindications to MRI are limited. Iron-containing intraocular foreign bodies, cochlear implants, and intracranial vascular clips can move and should not be exposed to the strong magnet. If an intraorbital foreign body is suspected, a limited CT scan of the orbit may be performed to ensure the safety of the MRI. Cardiac pacemakers may malfunction due to reprogramming of the unit. Some patients may not be able to withstand the claustrophobic conditions under which MRI is conducted, even with sedation.

COMPUTED TOMOGRAPHY

The technique for CT scanning was originated by Sir Godfrey Hounsfield at EMI (Electrical and Musical Industries) in England and led to his being awarded the Nobel prize for medicine in 1979. To understand this modality, it is necessary to begin with a brief review of x-ray and tomographic techniques.

1-2-1 Physical Principles

When an x-ray is transmitted through a substance, the beam is attenuated as a function of both the atomic number of the element (or the effective atomic number of a complex structure) and the concentration of substances forming the structure. In reality, it is the effective electron density that causes the attenuation. Increasing the energy of the x-ray leads to a decrease in attenuation. Conventional x-ray films are taken with the film alongside the patient and perpendicular to the beam. Most of the rays pass perpendicular to the film; some are scattered in other directions. Because of the thickness of the structures being filmed and the superimposition of these same structures, unwanted shadows are seen in addition to the desired image.

Tomography was invented to eliminate these undesired shadows and to concentrate on the object of interest. In this technique, the x-ray source and the film move relative to the patient during exposure. The point at which this x-ray source–film plane is pivoted is the object of interest. The desired structure remains motionless, and there is no relative movement between the film and the x-ray source.

1-2-2 Clinical Imaging Devices

Hounsfield's innovation was to use a computer to improve on the technique of tomography. Initially, only axial sections were obtainable; thus the previous term, *computerized axial tomography (CAT) scanning*. An assembly was created with the x-ray detector on one side of the object to be scanned rigidly connected to a collimated source of x-rays on the other side. This device, the gantry, allowed the x-ray tube and the detector to rotate around the patient as a single unit and permitted the angle of incoming x-rays to be altered, creating 180 images 1° apart. The computer could then reconstruct the image from the data points resulting from the attenuation of the x-ray beams. These data points were represented as pixels of a numeric value, based on the attenuation noted. This attenuation seen on the two-dimensional pixel is based on the three-dimensional voxel. The original EMI matrix was an acquisition pixel grid of 80×80, allowing for a voxel $3 \times 3 \times 13$ mm. Current scanners employ 512×512 or 1024×1024.

1-2-3 Windows

The attenuation coefficient was given an arbitrary value by Hounsfield: water was set at 0 and air at -500. On the original scale, dense bone had a typical value of $+500$. Subsequently, these values were doubled, creating Hounsfield units, abbreviated H, ranging from air at -1000 to bone at $+1000$. The importance of these numbers is in providing a numeric matrix from which the computer is able to yield a picture used for diagnostic purposes. The relationship of the attenuation coefficient to the entire gray scale can be displayed on a cathode-ray tube. The extremes of the scale can be modified so that differences of 1 unit or 100 units can be distinguished. This modification provides the window width, a function not possible on the conventional x-ray. This sets the scale between black and white. The window level is the central point of the window. This can be changed to emphasize different aspects of the scanned substance. A single film does not have enough range of gray scale to display all of the data in the computer (compare Figures 2-35 and 3-9). Thus, it may be necessary to split the data and display it on more than one film. In orbital scanning, both soft tissue and bone windows may be required to assess the extent of a lesion. A central soft tissue window level is usually near 0 to 40 H, with a width of 200 to 400 H. This allows for adequate contrast between fat and air. Bone windows may have a central level between 40 and 300 H, with a width of 2400 to 3200 H. This wide window width is necessary because of the variable density of bone.

1-2-4 Development of CT Technology

The accelerated development of the technology of computed tomographic scanning has led to new generations of advanced scanners. These have provided several advantages:

1. Decreased time required for the examination is most important with children and uncooperative patients. Instead of a single x-ray beam, a fan beam could be emitted and received by a number of detectors. Less imaging time also reduced motion artifact.

2. Increased resolution is obtained by decreasing voxel size through more rapid switching of the detectors. This allows for increased detail at no increased radiation risk. The dosage for a single emission is considerably less than that of a plain tomogram and is identical to that of a conventional x-ray, but is more focused to yield less diffuse radiation damage.

3. Thinner sections allow for increased detail with decreased background noise. This prevents partial volume averaging, a phenomenon wherein anatomic details are averaged across the depth of the section.

4. Larger gantry apertures make possible direct coronal scans and certain nonmidline sagittal scans.

1-2-5 Axial-Plane Imaging

The axial plane of sectioning is usually related to either the orbitomeatal line, OML, or Reid's anatomic baseline, RBL (Figure 1-25). OML is a straight line from the lateral canthus to the center of the external auditory meatus. RBL is a line between the inferior orbital rim and the upper margin of the external auditory meatus. This so-called anthropologic baseline is 10° negative to OML. An important angle is the plane of the optic canal, which is −10° to RBL and −20° to OML. Orbits are usually scanned parallel to RBL or 10° negative to OML to achieve an axial-plane angle parallel to the orbital floor. For intracranial structures, angulation between 0° and +25° to OML is useful, with less positively angulated images preferred for the sellar region, the middle range for the cerebral hemispheres, and the most positively angulated images for the posterior fossa.

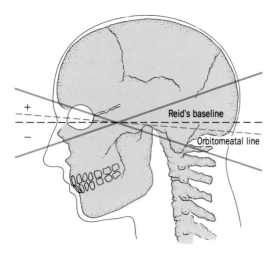

Reid's baseline

Orbitomeatal line

Figure 1-25 *Direction of the x-ray beam in the axial plane. The orbitomeatal line extends from the lateral canthus to the center of the external auditory meatus and is the reference plane for positive (+) and negative (−) angulation. Reid's anatomic baseline extends from the inferior orbital rim to the uper margin of the external auditory meatus. Axial head scans are performed with positive angulation and may include the medulla oblongata and the base of the frontal lobe on the lowest slice; the orbit will be missed. Axial orbit scans are performed with negative angulation. Separate orbit and head sequences are usually required.*

1-2-6 Coronal-Plane Imaging

Direct coronal scans require placing the patient in a prone position, with the head rested on the chin, or in a supine position, with the head extended back on its vertex. Coronal scans are taken at 90° angulation to RBL (Figure 1-26). Dental fillings may prevent direct coronal scans; the plane may need to be changed to avoid inducing artifact. The amount of deviation from the 90° axis must be individualized to provide as close to a direct coronal image as possible without artifact. Figure 1-27 shows the scout film for a coronal series in an edentulous patient. No compromise of angle was required, so that an almost true coronal plane was achieved.

Coronal reconstructions provide good anatomic information if axial scans are taken in ultrathin (1.5 mm) slices, exposing the patient to increased radiation doses. These images are still useful for a patient who cannot be placed in a direct coronal position, such as a young child, a comatose or elderly patient, and a trauma patient. Cross-sectional views of structures at right angles to the plane of the scan are particularly useful in orbital and parasellar scanning. Direct coronal images are better than axial images in assessing the inferior and superior rectus muscles, the orbital walls, the optic nerve, the optic chiasm, and other sellar and parasellar structures. In CT imaging, direct coronal scans are obtained with the patient in the prone position with the neck extended. The limitations of the CT gantry tilt angle do not allow the true coronal plane to be achieved, whereas MRI permits a true coronal scan to be achieved with the patient supine and without the neck extended.

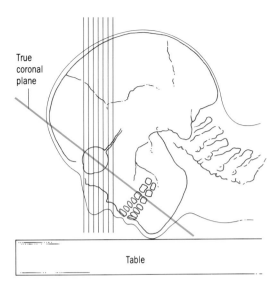

True
coronal
plane

Table

Figure 1-26 *Relative position of the head and the direction of the x-ray beam for direct coronal scanning of the orbit. Note that the neck scan cannot be extended sufficiently to achieve a true coronal plane. Moreover, the angulation may have to be further reduced from the direct coronal plane when the beam is directed anterior to the teeth to avoid artifacts from metallic fillings. Only MRI allows imaging in the true coronal plane.*

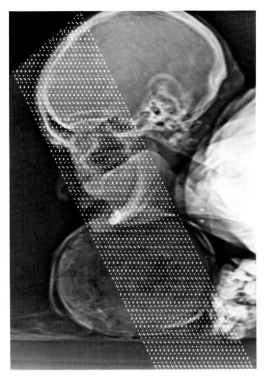

Figure 1-27 *A scout CT for an almost true direct coronal series of scans in an edentulous patient. No compromise of angle was required to avoid the metallic artifacts caused by dental fillings.*

1-2-7 Computer Analysis

CT scans can be oriented to slice or volume. Slice-oriented scanning uses single sections for diagnostic value. Thin sections and proper alignment of the plane of scanning are crucial to achieving maximal resolution. Volume-oriented scanning includes overlapping adjacent thicker sections, which allows for calculations of the volume of the orbit, globe, or rectus muscles. In addition, this technique is used in plastic and reconstructive surgery to create three-dimensional surface renderings of the bony orbit. Use of overlapping sections exposes the patient to increased radiation and causes more movement artifact.

1-2-8 Contrast Enhancement

Injection of intravenous contrast media is an adjunct to CT scanning. These dyes do not cross an intact blood–brain barrier. If the barrier is disturbed, however, concentration of the dye will be increased in the abnormal tissue. In the diagnosis of orbital disorders, abnormalities of the blood–brain barrier are rarely of clinical value. As a result, noncontrast scans are usually taken in this region. However, if intracranial extension of an orbital lesion is suspected, contrast enhancement may demonstrate it. In addition, contrast is crucial in the evaluation of chiasmal and parachiasmal lesions. The major complications following the use of contrast media are allergic reactions and can be life-threatening. The physician should be familiar with these problems and determine whether the patient has experienced any adverse reactions to seafood or iodine-containing contrast agents in the past.

1-2-9 X-Ray Dosage

Damage to the lens may occur in the infant at doses above 750 rads (cGy) and in the adult at doses above 2000 rads. Standard scanning techniques result in doses of about 3 to 5 rads in the scanned tissue, and high-resolution scanners may elevate the dosage to 10 rads.

1-3

ORDERING IMAGES

The specific indications for obtaining imaging in particular disease entities are beyond the scope of this volume. Images should be ordered after a complete history has been taken, a thorough examination performed, and a differential diagnosis entertained. In some conditions, several clinical examinations of the patient may be more valuable than obtaining imaging studies after the first visit. The better-defined the differential diagnosis, the more appropriate the imaging, enhancing the value of the scanning to the patient. Both MRI and CT techniques should be used for any situation where they may be complementary, and they should be extended or repeated if necessary to obtain the required information.

1-3-1 Selection of Technique

Choosing which type of scan to obtain, the area to scan, and whether to use contrast enhancement is crucial in obtaining maximal information from imaging procedures. Considerations include the seriousness of the condition, the potential for treating the condition once diagnosed, the urgency with which the scan must be obtained, and the cost-to-benefit ratio for the patient. CT scans are considerably less expensive than MRI scans and are usually adequate for many orbital studies. CT almost always provides better information than conventional x-ray plain films, which are often the community standard because of cost, insurance reimbursement, and scanner availability. In general, CT scans are performed in acute situations, especially trauma, where the possibility of a foreign body exists. If the presence of a metallic foreign body is suspected, a preliminary limited CT scan can rule out the possibility, allowing MRI to be performed.

CT is sufficient for imaging lacrimal gland tumors where the critical factors are the presence of the cortical bony indentation and remodeling of the lacrimal gland fossa with benign mixed tumor, as opposed to the irregular bone destruction and enhancing and nonenhancing regions characteristic of lacrimal gland carcinomas. Regional enhancement of lacrimal gland malignancies can also be seen with MRI. CT scans are used for the initial evaluation of disorders of the paranasal sinuses and for orbital fractures. Intraocular tumors can be evaluated with either CT or MRI. In cases of retinoblastoma, CT is useful for detecting calcium deposits within the tumor. MRI could be more helpful than CT for most other intraocular tumors, especially melanoma, which is paramagnetic. Optic nerve tumors will always require assessment of the intracanalicular and intracranial portions of the optic nerve so that MRI is preferred, although a CT to image the bony orbital apex may provide useful and complementary information. Most optic nerve inflammatory and demyelinating conditions are better imaged with MRI than CT. There are few intracranial conditions that are not best examined initially with MRI, except for acute intracranial hemorrhages or in patients for whom MRI is contraindicated.

If scanning a lesion will not make any difference in the treatment offered, the technique may not be necessary. Availability in the geographic location of one's practice is also a major consideration. The patient may benefit from undergoing a procedure that provides slightly less information if traveling hundreds of miles is not required. In addition, a scan performed at a great distance may be difficult to examine or discuss with the involved radiologist, creating problems in acute situations when scanned images are required in the operating room.

1-4

INTERPRETING IMAGES

As in other disciplines, interpreting CT and MRI scans requires practice and a systematic approach. It is important to review the preliminary data provided on the scan. This includes the patient's name and age, date of scan, technique performed, whether contrast enhancement was used, slice thickness, and right–left orientation. On CT images, the window width and center are provided and the order of scans is usually listed by image number. On MRI scans, TR, TE, and, with IR sequences, TI should be reviewed to assess the weighting of the image. In addition, the ACQ or NEX, matrix, and FOV are provided. Slice location is usually centered around a point designated as zero, with the initial scans shown as negative with regard to the zero position. Standard convention is to scan from inferior to superior in the axial plane, anterior to posterior in the coronal plane, and left to right in the sagittal plane. The sagittal-plane convention is the most variable as set by the manufacturer or operator. It is important to corroborate the assumed convention when the outcome is critical.

1-4-1 Examination of Images

After review of the identifying and acquisition information, attention is turned to the images themselves. It is important to orient oneself to the plane of scanning. This may be done by examining the scout film, which shows the slices as sectioned by the computer. Axial and coronal images can be confused if one is not familiar with the area of the brain being imaged.

Reviewing the information on the scans requires experience. It is necessary to examine bone, soft tissue, blood vessels, and CSF-containing structures to assess normality. Abnormalities can be represented by displacement; for example, a midline shift of the brain or a herniation of the brain stem down through the foramen magnum. Intensity of structures may be altered by pathology; often this can be seen best by comparing the two sides of the same patient. Look carefully for head rotation that can produce asymmetries of no diagnostic significance. Local areas of

signal alteration often represent abnormal deposition of materials such as melanin, calcium, or foreign bodies.

Misinterpretation of images often results when the necessary information could not be provided by the test performed. Examples include orbital floor fractures, where failure to perform direct coronal scans may cause the lesion to be missed, and meningiomas involving the optic nerve and cavernous sinus walls, lesions that are often difficult to recognize without—and even with—contrast enhancement. Often, scans are ordered to assess optic nerve pathology. However, the studies actually performed scan the brain and yield only one or two sections through the optic nerve, often at an inappropriate angulation. Within the orbit, difficulty arises with MRI techniques that produce chemical shift artifacts along the globe and optic nerve, mimicking pathology. These may require fat-suppression techniques to resolve.

1-4-2 Appearance of Intracranial Hemorrhage

The CT and MRI appearance of extravascular blood is of importance in evaluating the progression of hemorrhage into tissue as a result of disease processes, including trauma and tumors. CT is generally the best way to detect active or recent bleeding, especially when it is located in the cerebral ventricles or the subarachnoid space. CT also remains the preferred means for the initial emergent evaluation of suspected intracranial and orbital hemorrhage. Acute bleeding can be recognized on a non–contrast-enhanced CT. In addition, trauma patients benefit from the CT evaluation of fractures and the exclusion of the possible presence of magnetic foreign bodies. Nevertheless, MRI examination is becoming increasingly important in initial as well as followup examinations where CT does not give as much information as MRI concerning the location of subacute blood, the presence of aneurysms, and other diagnostic considerations. MRI can detect small hemorrhages, especially those in the posterior fossa that could be missed by CT due to bone artifact. Moreover, MR angiography is readily combined to give additional information concerning abnormal vessel configurations and thrombosed veins.

Acute intracerebral bleeding (less than 6 hours' duration) usually appears bright on CT scanning due to attenuation of the x-rays by hemoglobin. Subacute intraparenchymal blood is often isodense with brain on CT scans. In the chronic stage following bleeding (more than 2 weeks), intraparenchymal changes and loss of tissue cause the affected area to appear dark. The progression of intraparenchymal hemorrhage on MRI scanning is compared with that on CT in Table 1-3. Note that by the time of the subacute stage (approximately 1 week), MRI becomes the preferred method of examination.

SUGGESTED READINGS

Atlas SW: *Magnetic Resonance Imaging of the Brain and Spine.* New York: Raven Press; 1991.

Edelman RR, Hesselink JR: *Clinical Magnetic Resonance Imaging.* Philadelphia: WB Saunders Co; 1990.

Kretschmann H, Weinrich W: *Neuroanatomy and Computed Cranial Tomography.* New York: Thieme; 1986.

Latchaw RE: *MR and CT Imaging of the Head, Neck and Spine.* 2nd ed. St Louis: Mosby-Yearbook; 1991.

Mills CM, de Groot J, Posin JP: *Magnetic Resonance Imaging: Atlas of the Head, Neck and Spine.* Philadelphia: Lea & Febiger; 1988.

Newhouse J, Wiener J: *Understanding MRI.* Boston: Little, Brown & Co; 1991.

Osborne AG: *Handbook of Neuroradiology.* St Louis: CV Mosby Co; 1991.

Smith HJ, Ranallo FN: *A Non-Mathematical Approach to Basic MRI.* Madison: Medical Physics Publishing Corp; 1989.

CHAPTER 2

Globe and Orbit

GENERAL

2-1-1 MRI: Axial

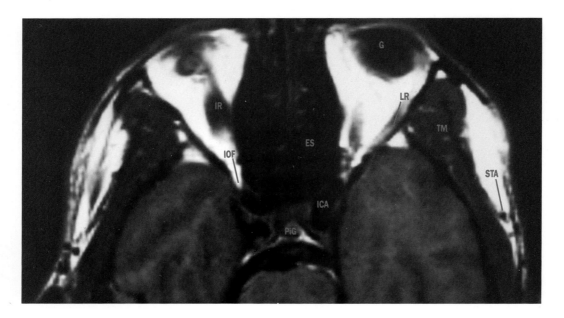

Figure 2-1 *T1-weighted, Inferior Rectus* This is the first and most inferior in a series of six negatively angled, axial, T1-weighted images taken at a slice thickness of 3 mm. Throughout, this atlas maintains the convention of starting all axial image series at the most inferior slice. On T1 weighting, the orbital fat is hyperintense and the vitreous and cerebrospinal fluid are hypointense. Portions of IR are seen bilaterally. The vertical recti are seen better on coronal and sagittal sections (compare Figures 2-13 and 2-22). It may be difficult to differentiate the inferior orbit from the superior without identifying adjacent structures such as the paranasal sinuses and the nasopharynx. These relationships are detailed in the section on sinus anatomy. The configuration of ES locates this section as being in the inferior orbit. IOF is labeled at the posterior limit of the hyperintense orbital fat. The fissure is hypointense and is immediately anterior to ICA in the cavernous sinus. Notice the neurovascular bundle lat-

ES	Ethmoid Sinus
G	Globe
ICA	Internal Carotid Artery
IOF	Inferior Orbital Fissure
IR	Inferior Rectus Muscle
LR	Lateral Rectus Muscle
PiG	Pituitary Gland
STA	Superficial Temporal Artery
TM	Temporalis Muscle

eral to TM. This bundle can be identified surgically in the fascia during surgery. It contains frontal branches of the facial nerve and STA.

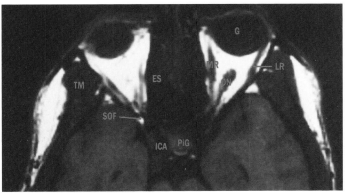

ES	Ethmoid Sinus
G	Globe
ICA	Internal Carotid Artery
LR	Lateral Rectus Muscle
MR	Medial Rectus Muscle
ON	Optic Nerve
PiG	Pituitary Gland
SOF	Superior Orbital Fissure
TM	Temporalis Muscle

Figure 2-2 *T1-weighted, Inferior Globe* This section is above the plane of the inferior rectus.

According to the convention followed throughout this atlas, the patient's left side is on the right side of the image. ON is the midline stucture on the left side. The posterior limit of the orbital fat marks SOF below the optic foramen. ICA creates the hypointense flow void lateral to PiG in each cavernous sinus.

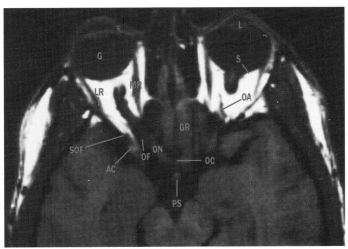

AC	Anterior Clinoid
G	Globe
GR	Gyrus Rectus of Frontal Lobe
L	Lens
LR	Lateral Rectus Muscle
MR	Medial Rectus Muscle
OA	Ophthalmic Artery
OC	Optic Chiasm
OF	Optic Foramen
ON	Optic Nerve
PS	Pituitary Stalk
S	Sclera
SOF	Superior Orbital Fissure

Figure 2-3 *T1-weighted, Midglobe* At this level, L can be seen bilaterally. ON extends through OF back to OC. SOF is seen lateral to the marrow of AC. MR is a larger structure than LR. MR is oriented in the anteroposterior plane parallel to the medial wall of the orbit. This is important when positioning an electromyography needle for chemodenervation of MR in cases of sixth-nerve palsy. OA is seen on the left, heading toward the medial wall of the orbit where its ethmoidal branches exit. OA follows a different course from the superior ophthalmic vein, which is seen in Figure 2-4. PS is seen posterior to OC, passing toward the pituitary gland (see Figure 2-2).

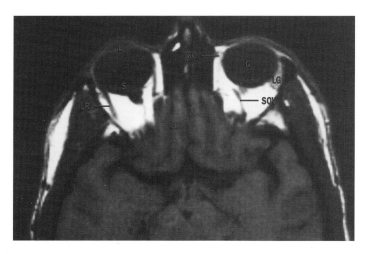

G	Globe
GR	Gyrus Rectus of Frontal Lobe
L	Lens
LG	Lacrimal Gland
LR	Lateral Rectus Muscle
S	Sclera
SO	Superior Oblique Muscle
SOV	Superior Ophthalmic Vein

Figure 2-4 *T1-weighted, Superior Globe* SOV is seen following its typical course from antero-medial to posterolateral in the orbit. Compare this to the course of the ophthalmic artery in Figure 2-3. SOV can be displaced, enlarged, or throm-bosed in various disease en-tities and is, therefore, an important structure to identify in orbital scans. The tendon of SO has passed through the trochlea and is heading for its insertion under the superior rectus muscle in the postero-lateral quadrant of the globe.

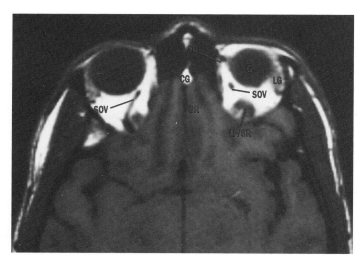

CG	Crista Galli of Ethmoid Bone
G	Globe
GR	Gyrus Rectus of Frontal Lobe
LG	Lacrimal Gland
LP	Levator Palpebrae Superioris
SO	Superior Oblique Muscle
SOV	Superior Ophthalmic Vein
SR	Superior Rectus Muscle

Figure 2-5 *T1-weighted, Lacrimal Gland* SOV is seen longitudi-nally on the right side and in cross section on the left. LG is located superolateral to G. CG is anterior to GR and is the an-terior attachment of the falx cerebri.

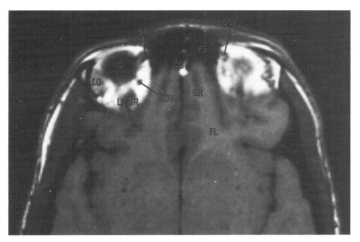

CG	Crista Galli of Ethmoid Bone
FL	Frontal Lobe
FS	Frontal Sinus
G	Globe
GR	Gyrus Rectus of Frontal Lobe
LG	Lacrimal Gland
LP	Levator Palpebrae Superioris
SO	Superior Oblique Muscle
SOV	Superior Ophthalmic Vein
SR	Superior Rectus Muscle

Figure 2-6 *T1-weighted, Levator Palpebrae Superioris and Superior Rectus* LP and SR cannot be separated and ap-pear to form one structure in the middle of the orbital roof. SOV is seen in cross section on the right side and longitudi-nally extending from its origin at the angular vein into the or-bit medially on the left side. FS is anterior to FL. At this level, the presence of FS and GR differentiate this view of the superior orbit from Figure 2-1, where the midline nasal structures identify the location as inferior orbit.

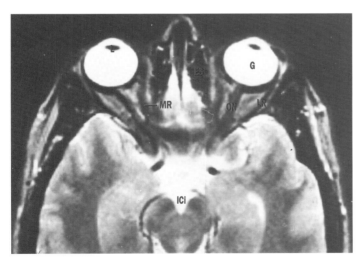

ES	Ethmoid Sinus
G	Globe
ICi	Interpeduncular Cistern
L	Lens
LR	Lateral Rectus Muscle
MR	Medial Rectus Muscle
ON	Optic Nerve

Figure 2-7 *T2-weighted, Midglobe* The bright signal produced by the water within G and cere-brospinal fluid cisterns charac-terize T2-weighted scans. The hyperintense signal of orbital fat in T1-weighted images makes it possible to differenti-ate the orbital muscles and vessels. The time required to obtain T2-weighted scans is greater than that required for T1-weighted scans and is long enough to produce undesirable motion artifact when patients move their eyes during scan-ning. Thus, T2-weighted images of the orbit are not frequently used in clinical practice.

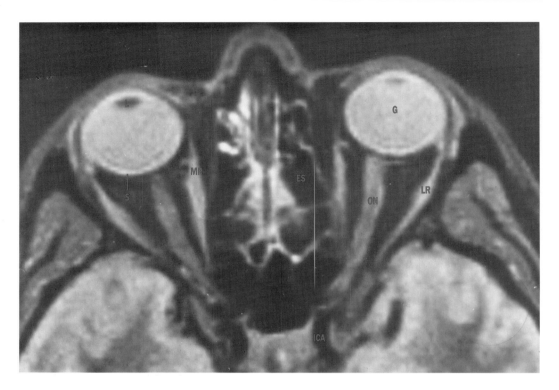

Figure 2-8 *Fat-Suppressed, Midglobe* The Short Tau Inversion Recovery (STIR) sequence is one type of fat-suppression technique. This enables suppression of the normal bright signal from orbital fat on T1-weighted images, which may interfere with the signal from adjacent muscles and the optic nerve. Each ON is seen grazing the lateral recess of the sphenoid sinus at the apex of the orbit where it leaves the plane of the section superiorly to enter the optic foramen. ICA marks the anterior limit of the cavernous sinus and abuts the location of the superior orbital fissure.

ES	Ethmoid Sinus
G	Globe
ICA	Internal Carotid Artery
L	Lens
LR	Lateral Rectus Muscle
MR	Medial Rectus Muscle
ON	Optic Nerve
S	Sclera

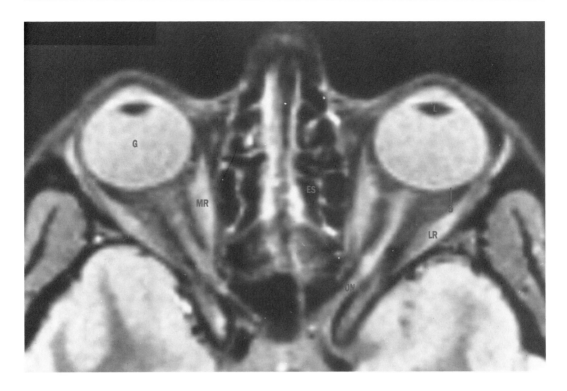

Figure 2-9 *Fat-Suppressed and Contrast-Enhanced, Midglobe*
The combination of fat suppression and contrast enhancement can reveal otherwise-undetectable optic nerve pathology. The right ON is normal as compared to ON on the left, which shows enhancement with contrast in its orbital portion. The abnormal portion of the left ON is hyperintense due to both the tissue changes and the use of contrast medium. This appearance is not diagnostic, but when accompanied by the appropriate clinical history supports a diagnosis of inflammatory optic neuropathy. The angulation of this image is slightly negative compared to Figure 2-8, showing the left ON passing through the optic foramen.

ES	Ethmoid Sinus
G	Globe
L	Lens
LR	Lateral Rectus Muscle
MR	Medial Rectus Muscle
ON	Optic Nerve
S	Sclera

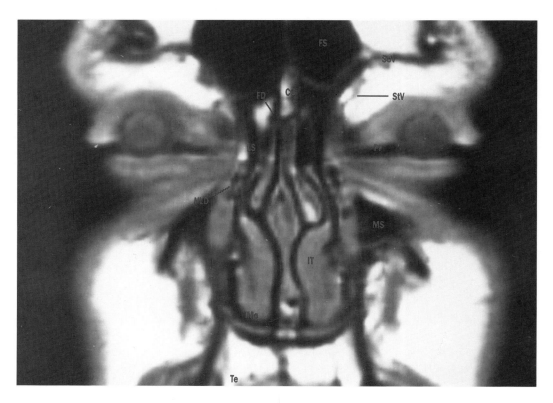

Figure 2-10 *T1-weighted, Lens*
Because most structures of neuro-ophthalmic interest extend longitudinally in the axial plane, coronal scans provide the opportunity to study them in cross section. MRI allows coronal scanning without repositioning the patient and thus enables imaging of patients who could not otherwise be imaged in the coronal plane, such as those with cervical spine disease. This figure is the most anterior of six scans in this series. Note the hyperintensity of the fat in the cheek, forehead, and skull marrow. Hyperintensity is also characteristic of the tooth-bearing aspects of the maxillary bone.

CG	Crista Galli of Ethmoid Bone
FD	Frontoethmoidal Duct
FS	Frontal Sinus
IMe	Inferior Meatus
IT	Inferior Turbinate
L	Lens
LS	Lacrimal Sac
MS	Maxillary Sinus
NLD	Nasolacrimal Duct
PF	Palpebral Fissure
SoV	Supraorbital Vessel
StV	Supratrochlear Vessel
Te	Teeth

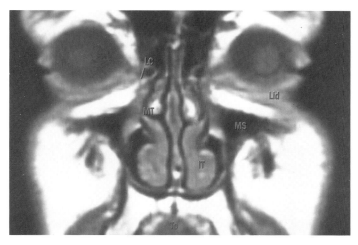

IT	Inferior Turbinate
LC	Lacrimal Canaliculus
Lid	Eyelid
MS	Maxillary Sinus
MT	Middle Turbinate
To	Tongue

Figure 2-11 *T1-weighted, Anterior to Midglobe* This slice is 3 mm posterior to that in Figure 2-10. Cartilage comprises the hyper-intense region within MT. The terms *concha* and *turbinate* are often confused. A concha is a bony structure; the inferior concha is a separate bone that forms the most inferomedial aspect of the bony nasolacrimal canal, while the superior and middle conchae are parts of the ethmoid bone. A turbinate is that portion of a concha covered by a mucous membrane. Thus, on bone window CT images the conchae are seen, while on MRI scans the turbinates are visualized. LC can be identified in the posterior aspect of Lid where it enters the nasolacrimal sac.

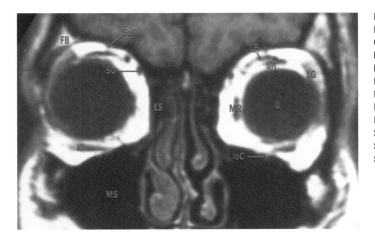

ES	Ethmoid Sinus
FB	Frontal Bone
G	Globe
IO	Inferior Oblique Muscle
IoC	Infraorbital Canal
LG	Lacrimal Gland
LP	Levator Palpebrae Superioris
MR	Medial Rectus Muscle
MS	Maxillary Sinus
SO	Superior Oblique Muscle
SoN	Supraorbital Notch
SR	Superior Rectus Muscle

Figure 2-12 *T1-weighted, Midglobe* The belly of SO is sectioned posterior to the trochlea. SR and LP can be distinguished as separate structures, with LP superior to SR. The aponeuro-sis of the left LP extends medially from the midline structure of LP. The origin of the right IO arises from the medial aspect of the inferior orbital rim.

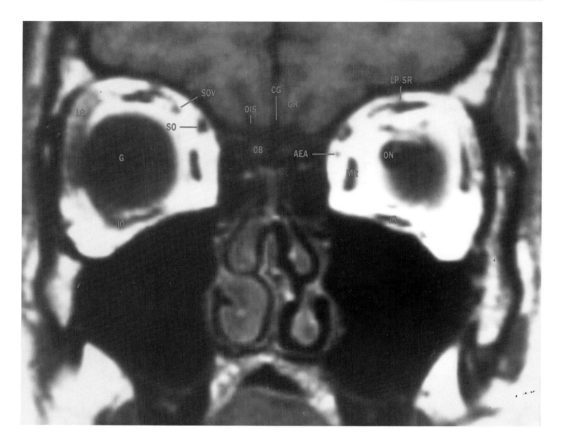

Figure 2-13 *T1-weighted, Posterior Globe* Coronal scans of the orbit may be helpful in making the diagnosis of dysthyroid ophthalmopathy by demonstrating enlargement of the extraocular muscles. AEA is seen between MR and SO heading toward its foramen at the frontoethmoidal suture. If the artery is severed near the medial wall during surgery, it may spring back into the orbital fat and bleed uncontrollably. OB may be the site of esthesioneuroblastoma, a tumor that may extend into the orbit. CG is a triangular process of the ethmoid bone growing upward from the cribriform plate to which the falx cerebri is attached. Orbital or lacrimal surgery may cause fractures of the cribriform plate.

AEA	Anterior Ethmoidal Artery
CG	Crista Galli of Ethmoid Bone
G	Globe
GR	Gyrus Rectus of Frontal Lobe
IO	Inferior Oblique Muscle
IR	Inferior Rectus Muscle
LG	Lacrimal Gland
LP	Levator Palpebrae Superioris
MR	Medial Rectus
OB	Olfactory Bulb
OIS	Olfactory Sulcus
ON	Optic Nerve
SO	Superior Oblique Muscle
SOV	Superior Ophthalmic Vein
SR	Superior Rectus Muscle

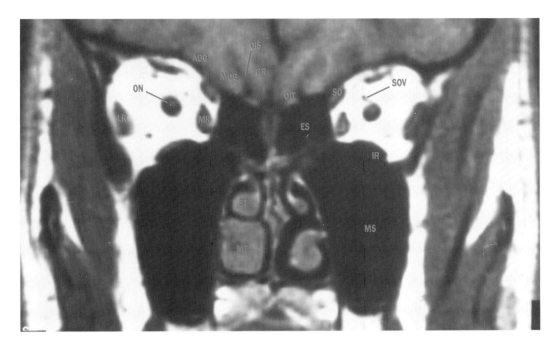

Figure 2-14 *T1-weighted, Posterior to Globe* This slice is 12 mm posterior to that in Figure 2-13. Coronal planes are often better than axial planes for viewing the optic nerves. Because of the tortuous course of the orbital optic nerve, axial sections often contain only a part of the nerve; whereas serial coronal scans demonstrate cross-sectional views. This image clearly shows the dark rim of cerebrospinal fluid within the dural sheath surrounding the lighter structure of ON (see also Figure 2-18). This view can be particularly helpful in differentiating enlargement of the substance of the nerve itself, as in optic gliomas, from enlargement of the sheath, as in optic nerve meningiomas. Meningiomas in the olfactory groove can arise from the dura surrounding OIT. These lesions cause the Foster Kennedy syndrome of unilateral optic atrophy, contralateral papilledema, and anosmia. The optic nervehead has a similar appearance in anterior ischemic optic neuropathy, a more common disorder causing pseudo–Foster Kennedy syndrome. Note that the top of MR is nearly at the level of GR, which lies above the cribriform plate of the ethmoid bone. MR is separated from GR by ES. Both surgical and nonsurgical trauma to the ethmoid and orbital regions may be associated with fractures of the cribriform plate that may lead to cerebrospinal fluid rhinorrhea and meningitis.

AOG	Anterior Orbital Gyrus
ES	Ethmoid Sinus
GR	Gyrus Rectus of Frontal Lobe
IR	Inferior Rectus Muscle
LR	Lateral Rectus Muscle
MOG	Medial Orbital Gyrus
MR	Medial Rectus Muscle
MS	Maxillary Sinus
MT	Middle Turbinate
OIS	Olfactory Sulcus
OIT	Olfactory Tract
ON	Optic Nerve
SO	Superior Oblique Muscle
SOV	Superior Ophthalmic Vein
ST	Superior Turbinate

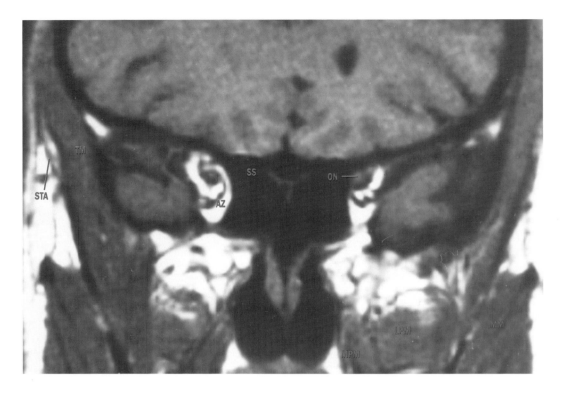

Figure 2-15 *T1-weighted, Orbital Apex* The superficial temporal veins and STA, along with frontal branches of the facial nerve, course through the fascial plane covering the fat lateral to TM. Frontalis muscle paralysis may result from failure to protect these nerves during lateral orbitotomy. AZ (also called the *common tendinous ring*) surrounds the optic foramen and part of the superior orbital fissure and consists of superior and inferior arching ligaments. The superior portion, the *upper tendon of Lockwood*, arises from the body of the sphenoid bone and gives rise to part of the lateral and

medial rectus muscles and the entirety of the superior rectus muscle. The inferior portion is called the *lower tendon of Zinn* and gives rise to the inferior rectus muscle, as well as parts of the medial and lateral rectus muscles. The portion of the superior orbital fissure that lies lateral to AZ contains (from top down) the lacrimal, frontal, and trochlear nerves. As a result, the trochlear nerve is usually not affected by retrobulbar anesthesia. TM and MM close the jaw, whereas LPM opens the jaw and its innervation (the motor branch of cranial nerve V) can be injured if TM is deeply retracted or cauterized during lateral orbitotomy.

AZ	Annulus of Zinn
LPM	Lateral Pterygoid Muscle
MM	Masseter Muscle
MPM	Medial Pterygoid Muscle
ON	Optic Nerve
SS	Sphenoid Sinus
STA	Superficial Temporal Artery
TM	Temporalis Muscle

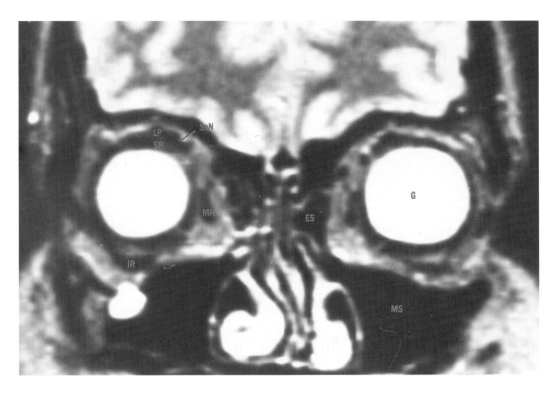

Figure 2-16 *T2-weighted, Midglobe*
This image demonstrates why T2-weighted images of the orbit are not frequently used in clinical practice (compare Figure 2-12). Without the bright signal produced by the orbital fat in T1-weighted images, it becomes more difficult to differentiate the orbital muscles and vessels. The time required to obtain T2-weighted scans is greater than that required for T1-weighted scans and is long enough to allow for motion artifact because patients move their eyes during scanning.

ES	Ethmoid Sinus
G	Globe
IR	Inferior Rectus Muscle
LP	Levator Palpebrae Superioris
MR	Medial Rectus Muscle
MS	Maxillary Sinus
SoN	Supraorbital Notch
SR	Superior Rectus Muscle

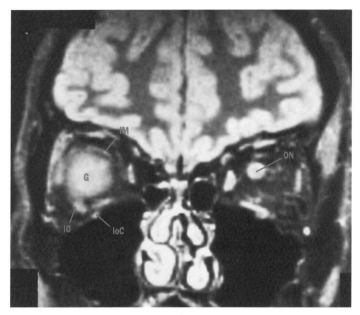

G	Globe
IM	Intermuscular Membrane
IO	Inferior Oblique Muscle
IoC	Infraorbital Canal
ON	Optic Nerve

Figure 2-17 *Fat-Suppressed, Posterior Globe and Optic Nerve* Both G and ON appear in this figure because the head is slightly rotated. This STIR image suppresses the orbital fat and augments the water signal of the extraocular muscles and the vitreous body. This technique also enhances the identification of IM and other connective tissue septae. The neurovascular bundle of the infraorbital nerve is seen in IoC.

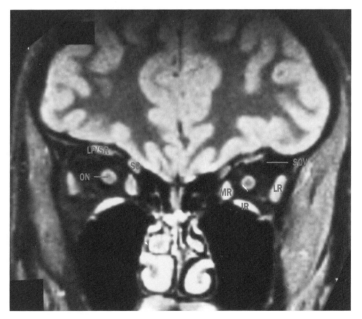

IR	Inferior Rectus Muscle
LP	Levator Palpebrae Superioris
LR	Lateral Rectus Muscle
MR	Medial Rectus Muscle
ON	Optic Nerve
SO	Superior Oblique Muscle
SOV	Superior Ophthalmic Vein
SR	Superior Rectus Muscle

Figure 2-18 *Fat-Suppressed, Posterior to Globe* The absence of fat signals within the orbit allows differentiation of the dural sheath of ON. The cerebrospinal fluid is seen as a bright ring surrounding the darker ON. The flow void of SOV is seen below the left SR.

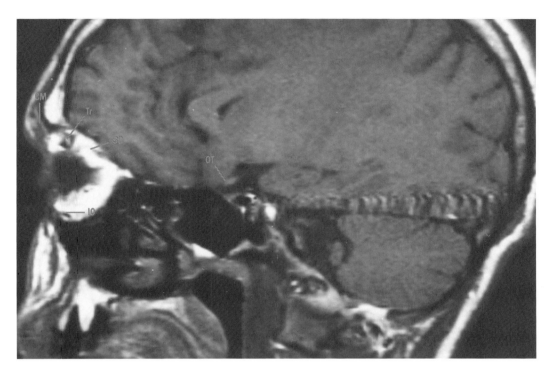

Figure 2-19 *T1-weighted, Trochlea*
This is the first of seven oblique parasagittal sections taken at a slice thickness of 3 mm, beginning at Tr and extending laterally through the lacrimal gland. The axis of the scan is 26° off the sagittal axis. This plane corresponds to the axis of the optic nerve and the vertical recti. It can be used for the examination of orbital floor fractures and may occasionally be useful for the examination of orbital tumors. The origin of IO is located in a shallow depression within the maxillary bone behind the in-ferior orbital rim and just lateral to the orifice of the naso-lacrimal canal. Tr is a curved fibrocartilaginous structure attached to the orbital surface of the frontal bone posterior to the orbital margin that creates a pulley through which the tendon of SO passes. Inflammation of or trauma involving Tr may produce a Brown's syndrome, with limited upgaze in adduction. Clinically, this must be differentiated by forced ductions from inferior oblique palsy. Except for IO, the comparative size of the right and left extraocular muscles is best seen on coronal scanning.

CM	Corrugator Muscle
IO	Inferior Oblique Muscle
OT	Optic Tract
SO	Superior Oblique Muscle
Tr	Trochlea

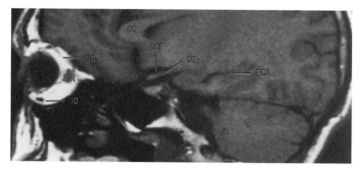

CC	Corpus Callosum
CCi	Crural Cistern
IO	Inferior Oblique Muscle
MR	Medial Rectus Muscle
OT	Optic Tract
PCA	Posterior Cerebral Artery
PH	Pes Hippocampus
SO	Superior Oblique Muscle

Figure 2-20 *T1-weighted, Lateral to Trochlea* SO is seen proximal to the trochlea. Intracranially, OT passes through CCi above PH. Because this is an oblique parasagittal section, only the genu of CC is seen (compare midline sagittal section, Figure 4-36). The oculomotor nerve is not seen here, within the interpeduncular cistern. It is usually better delineated in routinely angulated parasagittal images.

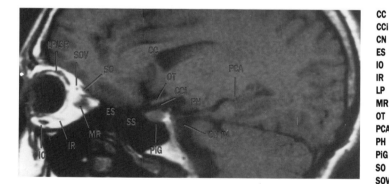

CC	Corpus Callosum
CCi	Crural Cistern
CN IV	Trochlear Nerve
ES	Ethmoid Sinus
IO	Inferior Oblique Muscle
IR	Inferior Rectus Muscle
LP	Levator Palpebrae Superioris
MR	Medial Rectus Muscle
OT	Optic Tract
PCA	Posterior Cerebral Artery
PH	Pes Hippocampus
PiG	Pituitary Gland
SO	Superior Oblique Muscle
SOV	Superior Ophthalmic Vein
SR	Superior Rectus Muscle
SS	Sphenoid Sinus

Figure 2-21 *T1-weighted, Origin of Superior Oblique* SO originates from the body of the sphenoid bone medial to the upper tendon of Lockwood and between the superior and medial recti. SOV is seen both in cross section and longitudinally as it drains toward the superior orbital fissure. This longitudinal section corresponds to the cross-sectional view of SOV seen in the axial section, Figure 2-5. ES is medial to the posterior orbit and adjacent to the optic foramen. LP and SR are adjacent structures and cannot be seen separately in this section.

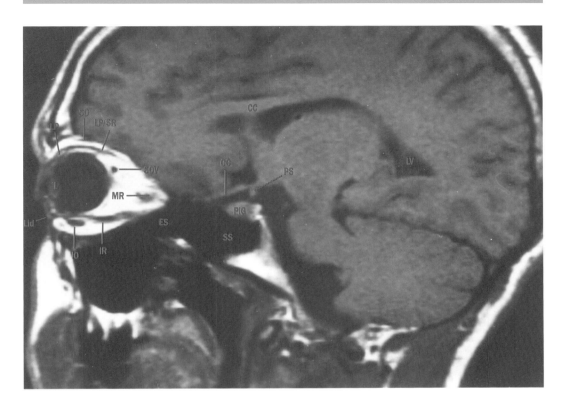

Figure 2-22 *T1-weighted, Midglobe*
The aponeurosis of LP extends forward and downward from Whitnall's transverse ligament (not visualized), which suspends the upper eyelid. LP and SR cannot be separated more posteriorly. IO crosses below IR at the suspensory ligament of Lockwood. The lower eyelid retractors extend anteriorly from the suspensory ligament of Lockwood into the orbital septum and tarsus of the lower eyelid. The trigone of LV is at the junction of the occipital and temporal horns with the body of LV.

CC	Corpus Callosum
ES	Ethmoid Sinus
IO	Inferior Oblique Muscle
IR	Inferior Rectus Muscle
L	Lens
Lid	Eyelid
LP	Levator Palpebrae Superioris
LV	Lateral Ventricle
MR	Medial Rectus Muscle
OC	Optic Chiasm
PiG	Pituitary Gland
PS	Pituitary Stalk
SO	Superior Oblique Muscle
SOV	Superior Ophthalmic Vein
SR	Superior Rectus Muscle
SS	Sphenoid Sinus

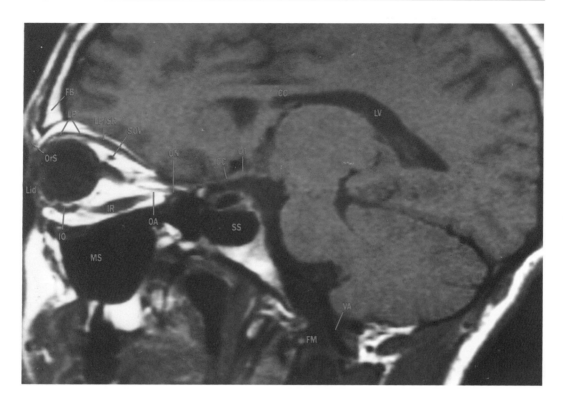

Figure 2-23 *T1-weighted, Optic Foramen* This parasagittal section permits a view of the most anterior portion of the visual pathway from the intraorbital ON through OC and the contralateral OT. Note that ON appears less intense in the orbit than does OT in the crural cistern. The tissues should have the same density, but the surrounding bright orbital fat makes ON appear darker. This section is useful for evaluating lesions of ON, particularly in the optic foramen. OA emerges from the optic foramen within the muscle cone and below ON. This view permits visualization of defects in the floor of the orbit that allow decompression into MS for Graves' disease or visualization of orbital floor fractures. This image illustrates the transantral approach through MS to the inferior orbit. The apex of the orbit cannot be directly decompressed by removing the roof of MS because its posterior wall terminates anterior to the apex. VA enters FM, passing over a groove on the posterior arch of the atlas.

CC	Corpus Callosum
FB	Frontal Bone
FM	Foramen Magnum
IO	Inferior Oblique Muscle
IR	Inferior Rectus Muscle
Lid	Eyelid
LP	Levator Palpebrae Superioris
LV	Lateral Ventricle
MS	Maxillary Sinus
OA	Ophthalmic Artery
OC	Optic Chiasm
ON	Optic Nerve
OrS	Orbital Septum
OT	Optic Tract
SOV	Superior Ophthalmic Vein
SR	Superior Rectus Muscle
SS	Sphenoid Sinus
VA	Vertebral Artery

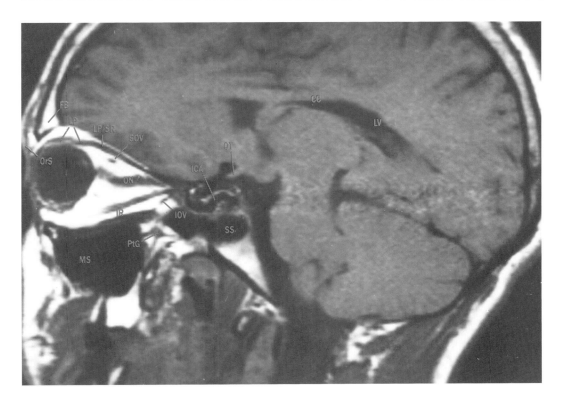

Figure 2-24 *T1-weighted, Intraorbital Optic Nerve* The eyelid contains OrS, often recognizable if defined by preaponeurotic fat, which is more prominent if the patient is elderly or obese. OrS extends down into the upper eyelid from the superior orbital rim of FB. ON follows a tortuous course within the orbit; the distance between the back of the globe and the anterior opening of the optic foramen is about 17 mm, while the length of the nerve is about 24 to 30 mm. IOV passes inferior to the muscle cone and drains via either the superior orbital fissure or the inferior orbital fissure into the cavernous sinus. PtG is seen posterior to MS in the pterygopalatine fossa. The S-shaped course of ICA marks the location of the cavernous sinus.

CC	Corpus Callosum
FB	Frontal Bone
ICA	Internal Carotid Artery
IOV	Inferior Ophthalmic Vein
IR	Inferior Rectus Muscle
LP	Levator Palpebrae Superioris
LV	Lateral Ventricle
MS	Maxillary Sinus
ON	Optic Nerve
OrS	Orbital Septum
OT	Optic Tract
PtG	Pterygopalatine Ganglion
SOV	Superior Ophthalmic Vein
SR	Superior Rectus Muscle
SS	Sphenoid Sinus

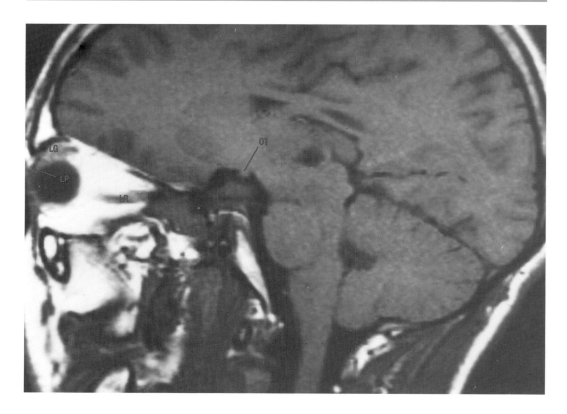

Figure 2-25 *T1-weighted, Lacrimal Gland* LG is divided into palpebral and orbital portions by the lateral horn of LP and is seen folded around LP in this image.

LG	Lacrimal Gland
LP	Levator Palpebrae Superioris
LR	Lateral Rectus Muscle
OT	Optic Tract

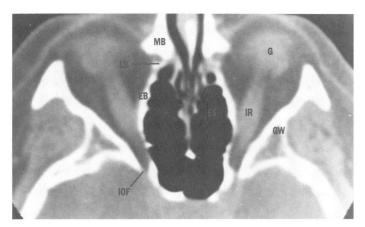

EB	Ethmoid Bone
ES	Ethmoid Sinus
G	Globe
GW	Greater Wing of Sphenoid Bone
IOF	Inferior Orbital Fissure
IR	Inferior Rectus Muscle
LB	Lacrimal Bone
MB	Maxillary Bone

Figure 2-26 *Inferior Rectus* This is the first of six axial CT scans of the orbit taken at different heights and angulations. Prior to interpretation of a scan, the angulation must be determined by identifying the most anterior and the most posterior structures in each image. CT offers the ability to readily define the bony fissures and foramina. The presence of a vertically acting rectus muscle indicates that the section is in the inferior or superior orbit. The medial walls are parallel to each other in the midorbit, where they extend in the sagittal plane. In the superior orbit, the posterior part of the medial wall again deviates laterally, causing the orbit to appear triangular or even quadrangular in the highest sections (Figures 2-30 and 2-31). IR can be seen in its entirety in this section because the angulation of the slice is negative. The frontal process of MB and the posterior lacrimal crest of LB form the boundaries of the bony nasolacrimal canal. The anterior air cells of ES extend to the level of the posterior lacrimal crest of the right side, but not the left in this section. The most anterior air cells of ES may extend anteriorly into the frontal process of MB. Knowledge of the variations in this anatomic relationship is helpful in performing a dacryo- cystorhinostomy (DCR) because opening the medial wall of the lacrimal sac fossa may lead first into the interposed ES and its mucosa before further penetrating the nasal cavity. IOF is located at the posterior medial wall of the orbit. Note the squamozygomatic surface of GW in the depth of the temporal fossa. The density of the bone at this location produces the oblique innominate line extending through the lateral orbit seen on conventional posteroanterior skull films (see Figures 2-39 and 2-40).

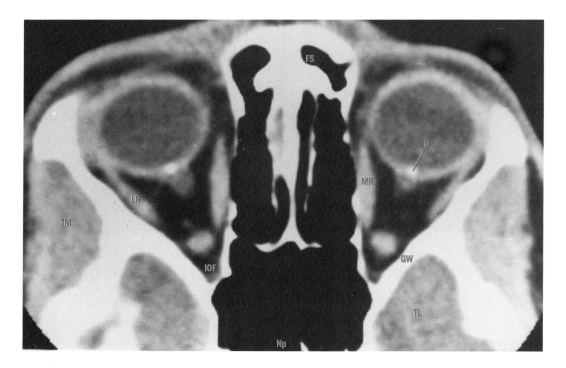

Figure 2-27 *Midglobe* Although this section includes the midglobe, it does not include the optic foramen. Because of the positive angulation, Np and IOF are seen posteriorly. The belly of TM appears largest in the lowest axial sections of the orbit and decreases in size in the higher sections. The muscle belly of MR is thickest at midorbit. Comparison of MR width with the diameter of the globe can give information about absolute enlargement of muscle in Graves' disease and orbital pseudotumor. D can be seen because of calcification, often as an incidental finding. LR is smaller than MR. The anterior portion of LR is separated from the lateral orbital wall by the hypodense orbital fat, which creates natural contrast in the orbit. Contrast enhancement is ordered for orbital scans only when it is desired to intensify vascular structures or tumors. TL occupies the middle cranial fossa and is separated from the orbit by GW. Defects of the posterior wall of the orbit can cause pulsatile exophthalmos in neurofibromatosis.

D	Drusen of Optic Nervehead
FS	Frontal Sinus
GW	Greater Wing of Sphenoid Bone
IOF	Inferior Orbital Fissure
LR	Lateral Rectus Muscle
MR	Medial Rectus Muscle
Np	Nasopharynx
TL	Temporal Lobe
TM	Temporalis Muscle

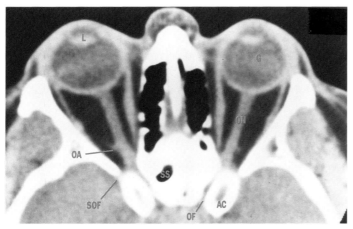

AC	Anterior Clinoid
G	Globe
L	Lens
OA	Ophthalmic Artery
OF	Optic Foramen
ON	Optic Nerve
SOF	Superior Orbital Fissure
SS	Sphenoid Sinus

Figure 2-28 *Midglobe Through Optic Foramen* This 3-mm section was obtained with optimal negative angulation to show both the midglobe and OF. Compare with Figure 2-45 with positive angulation, which shows only SOF. The presence of the suprasellar structures and the absence of the nasopharynx also serve to identify the negative angulation. On thicker sections, the partial volumes of the voxels containing ON and the superior rectus and levator palpebrae super-ioris muscles may combine to create the false impression that ON is enlarged by tumor. Identification of relevant structures will overcome this problem. ON may appear thickened by tumors, increased intracranial pressure causing enlargement of its sheaths, or inflammation. Atrophy or hypoplasia may cause the nerve to appear small, but caution should be exercised in making this interpretation from axial sections alone, without the benefit of coronal sections. Axial sections may contain only a partial volume of ON in the plane of section. The normal anteroposterior measurement of G is 50% to 55% of anteroposterior orbit measurement (cornea to anterior margin of OF). The diameters of G cannot be compared; nor can exophthalmos be measured on the axial view if the globes are scanned at different levels due to vertical displacement or tilt of the head. SS is shown surrounded by the body of the sphenoid bone. OF is only about 3 mm in diameter in comparison with SOF, which is about 3 cm in height. Superiorly, SOF flanks OF on the lateral side, from which it is separated by AC. Inferiorly, SOF lies directly below OF, allowing the larger structure to be confused for the smaller one in positively angled scans.

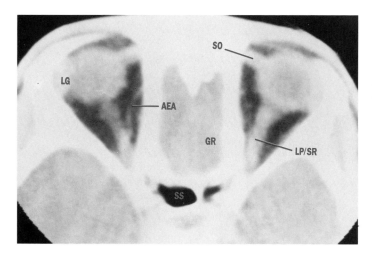

AEA	Anterior Ethmoidal Artery
GR	Gyrus Rectus of Frontal Lobe
LG	Lacrimal Gland
LP	Levator Palpebrae Superioris
SO	Superior Oblique Muscle
SR	Superior Rectus Muscle
SS	Sphenoid Sinus

Figure 2-29 *Superior Globe and Lacrimal Gland* The positive angulation of the section can be identified because SS is included in the section. The presence of GR between the almost parallel walls of the orbits helps to identify this as a superior orbital section. GR lies above the cribriform plate of the ethmoid bone. SO tendon is seen extending from the region of the trochlea to the equator of the globe. LG is denser than the surrounding orbital fat, so that it is naturally contrasted. Contrast media slightly enhance the normal LG, but may provide even more enhancement if the structure is involved by tumor or inflammation. The superior ophthalmic vein is usually seen in sections at this level (see Figure 2-43).

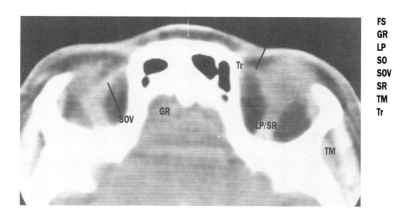

FS	Frontal Sinus
GR	Gyrus Rectus of Frontal Lobe
LP	Levator Palpebrae Superioris
SO	Superior Oblique Muscle
SOV	Superior Ophthalmic Vien
SR	Superior Rectus Muscle
TM	Temporalis Muscle
Tr	Trochlea

Figure 2-30 *Superior Rectus and Levator Palpebrae Superioris* SO and SR blend together at their insertions on the superior surface of the globe. SO inserts inferiorly to the insertion of SR. LP and SR form a wide band on this axial section and should not be confused with a thickened optic nerve.

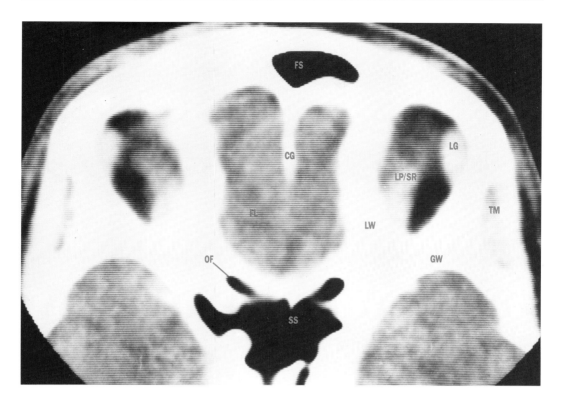

Figure 2-31 *Orbital Roof* This axial section is taken at a more positive angulation than the others in this series. The angle can be recognized because SS and OF are included in the posterior portion of the image. The gyrus rectus of FL is medial to the orbit. SR and LP are seen as a single structure in this slice. LP is located supero-laterally to SR and is the wider muscle. The origin of TM is seen at the superior margin of the temporal fossa. Axial sections such as this often appear as the only orbital view in a routine axial series of the head. A bony defect containing soft tissue at the orbital roof could suggest a frontal sinus mucopyocele or a meningoencephalocele extending into the orbit. Both of these conditions would be better evaluated with a coronal study.

CG	Crista Galli of Ethmoid Bone
FL	Frontal Lobe
FS	Frontal Sinus
GW	Greater Wing of Sphenoid Bone
LG	Lacrimal Gland
LP	Levator Palpebrae Superioris
LW	Lesser Wing of Sphenoid Bone
OF	Optic Foramen
SR	Superior Rectus Muscle
SS	Sphenoid Sinus
TM	Temporalis Muscle

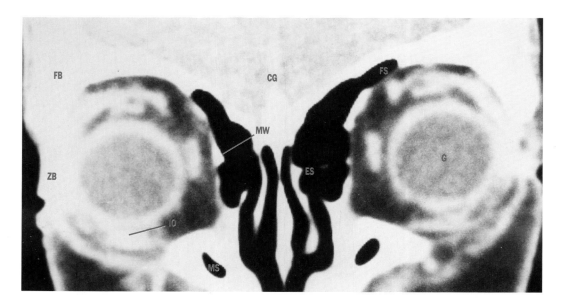

Figure 2-32 *Midglobe* In coronal sections of the orbit, the beam must pass anterior to the teeth if they contain metallic fillings (see Figure 1-26). Therefore, they will not be true coronal projections. G lies closer to the lateral wall than to MW. The coronal view is necessary to see vertical displacement of G. MW (or lamina papyracea) is the thin lateral wall of ES. MS appears small because this slice passes through its most anterior aspect. The origin and body of IO blend with the distal portion of the inferior rectus. Basal meningoencephaloceles can be recognized directly invading the superomedial orbit or indirectly invading the orbit via ES on coronal sections. This condition may be associated with congenital optic disc anomalies, such as optic nerve hypoplasia, coloboma, or megalopapilla. Medial encephaloceles are seen clinically just inferior to the medial canthal tendon and may be confused with congenital dacryoceles.

CG	Crista Galli of Ethmoid Bone
ES	Ethmoid Sinus
FB	Frontal Bone
FS	Frontal Sinus
G	Globe
IO	Inferior Oblique Muscle
MS	Maxillary Sinus
MW	Medial Wall of Orbit
ZB	Zygomatic Bone

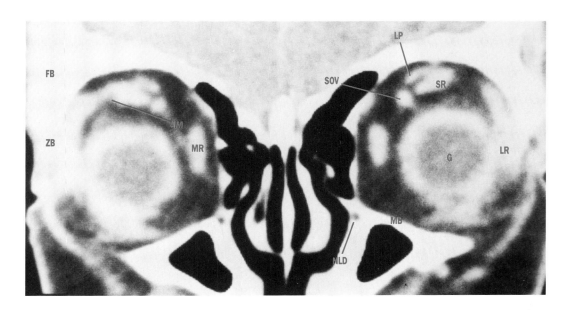

Figure 2-33 *Posterior Globe* In this slice, LR blends with IM and the lacrimal gland and is not seen as a distinct structure. IM joins all four rectus muscles, but is seen best in the superotemporal quadrant. SR is seen as a separate structure, inferior to LP (see Figure 2-34). NLD is seen within the bony nasolacrimal canal of MB.

FB	Frontal Bone
G	Globe
IM	Intermuscular Membrane
LP	Levator Palpebrae Superioris
LR	Lateral Rectus Muscle
MB	Maxillary Bone
MR	Medial Rectus Muscle
NLD	Nasolacrimal Duct
SOV	Superior Ophthalmic Vein
SR	Superior Rectus Muscle
ZB	Zygomatic Bone

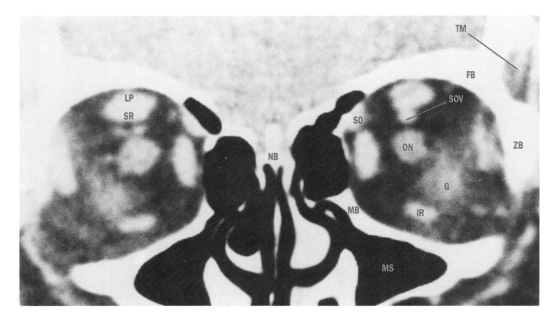

Figure 2-34 *Posterior to Globe* SO runs in the superomedial aspect of the orbit. SR and LP can no longer be separated from one another. Note that both G and ON are seen in the same slice, demonstrating that ON does not arise from the most posterior aspect of the globe. This direct coronal view is the optimal view for assessing blowout fractures of the medial wall and floor of the orbit. Unlike the Waters view obtained with conventional x-rays, CT allows visualization of the fracture as well as the location of IR, not just soft tissue prolapse into MS. Fractures of MB are usually described based on the Le Fort classification. Le Fort I fractures do not involve the orbit. Le Fort II midfacial fractures cause floor fractures and are the most common of the Le Fort fractures, occurring in 35% to 55% of maxillary fractures. By definition, the type II fracture passes through NB, across the frontal process of MB and the lacrimal bones, and descends through the infraorbital rim and into the lateral inferior wall of MS.

FB	Frontal Bone
G	Globe
IR	Inferior Rectus Muscle
LP	Levator Palpebrae Superioris
MB	Maxillary Bone
MS	Maxillary Sinus
NB	Nasal Bone
ON	Optic Nerve
SO	Superior Oblique Muscle
SOV	Superior Ophthalmic Vein
SR	Superior Rectus Muscle
TM	Temporalis Muscle
ZB	Zygomatic Bone

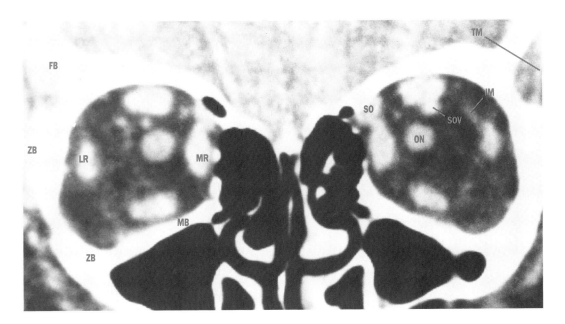

Figure 2-35 *Anterior to Orbital Apex* IM is less dense than in more anterior sections. MR and SO blend together (compare with Figure 2-34). SOV is larger than the more medially located branches of the ophthalmic artery. Le Fort III fractures represent a separation of the facial skeleton from the cranium. The orbital portion of this injury passes posterior to the inferior orbital fissure and divides into two lines. One line extends across the lateral wall near the sphenozygomatic junction, resulting in fronto-zygomatic disjunction with continuation inferiorly to separate the zygomatic arch, a so-called tripod fracture. The second line descends across the posterior MB to fracture the pterygoid plates of the sphenoid bone near the basisphenoid. If present, a tripod fracture would be well demonstrated on this section as lateral and inferior displacement of ZB. ZB forms the anterolateral portion of the orbital floor. TM is removed from FB during a lateral orbitotomy.

FB	Frontal Bone
IM	Intermuscular Membrane
LR	Lateral Rectus Muscle
MB	Maxillary Bone
MR	Medial Rectus Muscle
ON	Optic Nerve
SO	Superior Oblique Muscle
SOV	Superior Ophthalmic Vein
TM	Temporalis Muscle
ZB	Zygomatic Bone

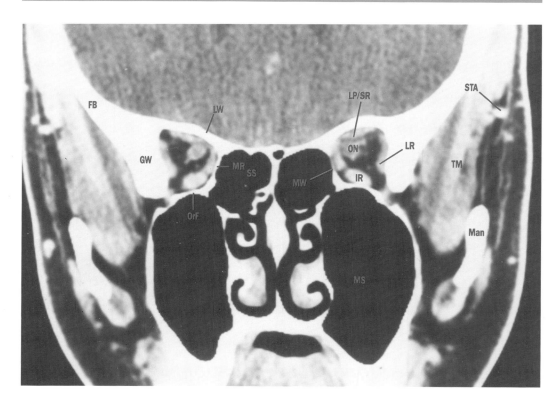

Figure 2-36 *Orbital Apex* The fascia surrounding TM is split into two layers covered with fat. STA and frontal branches of the facial nerve pass through this fascia en route to the frontalis muscle. At this window setting, an artifact is created whereby MS appears continuous with SS. Compare this with Figure 3-10, where a bone window shows the actual limits of these sinuses. Traumatic injuries may produce bony fragments in the optic foramen. Look for evidence of optic nerve trauma when blood is seen in SS or the posterior ethmoid sinuses.

FB	Frontal Bone
GW	Greater Wing of Sphenoid Bone
IR	Inferior Rectus Muscle
LP	Levator Palpebrae Superioris
LR	Lateral Rectus Muscle
LW	Lesser Wing of Sphenoid Bone
Man	Mandible
MR	Medial Rectus Muscle
MS	Maxillary Sinus
MW	Medial Wall of Orbit
ON	Optic Nerve
OrF	Orbital Floor
SR	Superior Rectus Muscle
SS	Sphenoid Sinus
STA	Superficial Temporal Artery
TM	Temporalis Muscle

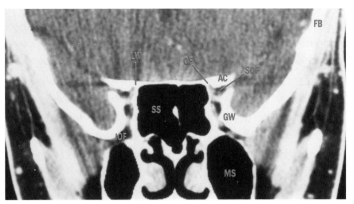

AC	Anterior Clinoid
FB	Frontal Bone
GW	Greater Wing of Sphenoid Bone
IOF	Inferior Orbital Fissure
LW	Lesser Wing of Sphenoid Bone
MS	Maxillary Sinus
OF	Optic Foramen
SOF	Superior Orbital Fissure
SS	Sphenoid Sinus

Figure 2-37 *Posterior Orbital Apex* The apex of the orbit can be conceived of as a triangular structure made up of its superior, medial, and lateral walls (compare with Figure 2-36, which is 20 mm anterior). The inferior wall does not extend as far posteriorly as the other three walls. As a result, a transantral (Caldwell-Luc) approach to the orbit does not allow access to OF. Continuity between SOF and IOF is well demonstrated here. SOF is situated between GW and LW. IOF lies between GW laterally and the palatine, maxillary, and zygomatic bones inferiorly and forms the boundary between the lateral and inferior walls of the orbit.

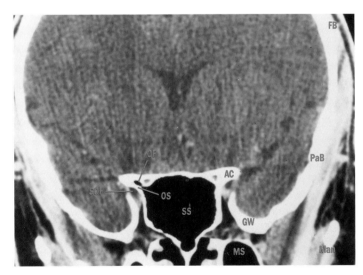

AC	Anterior Clinoid
FB	Frontal Bone
GW	Greater Wing of Sphenoid Bone
Man	Mandible
MS	Maxillary Sinus
OF	Optic Foramen
OS	Optic Strut of Sphenoid Bone
PaB	Parietal Bone
SOF	Superior Orbital Fissure
SS	Sphenoid Sinus

Figure 2-38 *Orbital Apex and Anterior Clinoid* OF within the lesser wing of the sphenoid bone is bounded inferolaterally by OS, which separates OF from SOF. Erosion of OS occurs with expansile lesions such as intracavernous aneurysms of the carotid artery. At midcanal, OF has a round configuration. More anteriorly, it forms a vertical ellipse, whereas posteriorly it forms a horizontal ellipse. Compare this soft tissue view with a bone window CT (Figure 3-10).

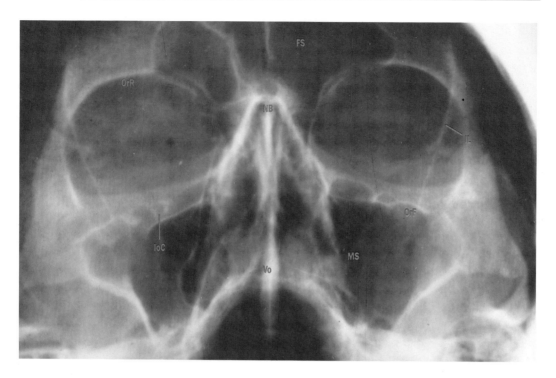

Figure 2-39 *Waters View* The Waters view is a posteroanterior film imaged with the head extended so that the cantho-meatal line lies at 37° to the central beam. The chin touches the film, and the nose is placed a variable distance away from the film depending on the facial configuration. Because this view projects the petrous temporal bone below the maxillary antrum, MS can be visualized. Fracture displacement of OrF into MS can be seen. However, while plain films may suggest facial fractures, CT scanning should be performed because it provides superior contrast resolution and detects concomitant intracranial injuries. OrR is seen clearly, making this a good view for seeing destruction of this bone, as in mucoceles of FS. This view can be extended to a 45° angle (exaggerated Waters view) to show the foramen magnum or reduced to 25° (modified Waters view) to demonstrate the foramen rotundum.

FS	Frontal Sinus
IL	Innominate Line
IoC	Infraorbital Canal
MS	Maxillary Sinus
NB	Nasal Bone
OrF	Orbital Floor
OrR	Orbital Roof
Vo	Vomer

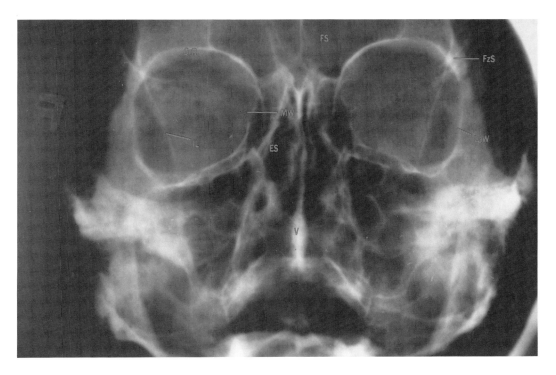

Figure 2-40 *Caldwell View* The Caldwell view is a posteroanterior film shot with the central x-ray beam positively angled 25° from the canthomeatal line toward the feet. The face is positioned with the forehead and nose touching the film. This enables better visualization of the superior and lateral orbital rims, FS, and ES. Note how indistinct the orbital floor and maxillary sinus are, compared to the Waters view seen in Figure 2-39. IL is seen running diagonally in the lateral third of the orbit. It represents the point of greatest density of the greater wing of the sphenoid bone. Agenesis or destruction of this bone (as in neurofibromatosis) may lead to the disappearance of IL. Occasionally, a large vein can be identified as a round defect immediately medial to IL; this is a normal anatomic variant.

ES	Ethmoid Sinus
FS	Frontal Sinus
FzS	Frontozygomatic Suture
IL	Innominate Line
LaW	Lateral Wall of Orbit
MW	Medial Wall of Orbit
OrR	Orbital Roof
Vo	Vomer

ORBITAL VESSELS

2-2-1 CT: Axial, Contrast-Enhanced

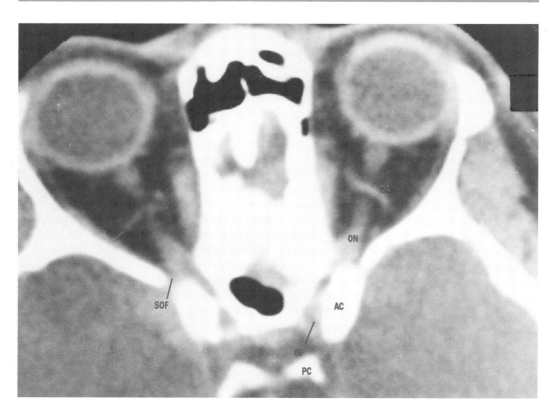

Figure 2-41 *Ophthalmic Artery* This slice shows both SOF and OF. If the slice does not contain AC, it is difficult to be absolutely sure that OF is visualized. SOF is at least 10 times the size of OF; thus, if one foramen is seen, it is likely to be SOF. Notice OA crossing over ON from lateral to medial. See Figure 2-3 for the MRI appearance of OA.

AC	Anterior Clinoid
OA	Ophthalmic Artery
OF	Optic Foramen
ON	Optic Nerve
PC	Posterior Clinoid
SOF	Superior Orbital Fissure

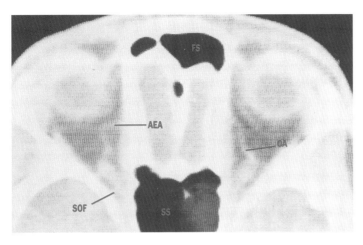

AEA Anterior Ethmoidal Artery
FS Frontal Sinus
OA Ophthalmic Artery
SOF Superior Orbital Fissure
SS Sphenoid Sinus

Figure 2-42 *Ophthalmic and Anterior Ethmoidal Arteries* Compare this with Figure 2-41. Here the angulation is more positive, the posterior orbit is sectioned more inferiorly, and the anterior orbit is sectioned more superiorly. OA crosses over the optic nerve from lateral to medial, and originates AEA, which passes between the superior oblique and medial rectus muscles en route to the anterior ethmoidal foramen about 15 mm posterior to the anterior lacrimal crest. The posterior ethmoidal foramen is about 35 mm posterior to the orbital rim. If AEA is severed during orbital surgery or trauma, it may spring back into the orbit and cause uncontrollable bleeding. The foramina for the anterior and posterior ethmoidal arteries are situated at the junction of the ethmoid and frontal bones and mark the border between the medial wall and the roof of the orbit.

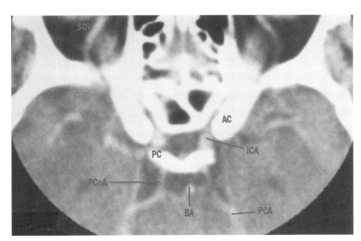

AC Anterior Clinoid
BA Basilar Artery
ICA Internal Carotid Artery
PC Posterior Clinoid
PCA Posterior Cerebral Artery
PCoA Posterior Communicating Artery
SOV Superior Ophthalmic Vein

Figure 2-43 *Superior Ophthalmic Vein* SOV lies in the superior aspect of the orbit and follows a characteristic course from anteromedial to posterolateral just below the superior rectus/levator palpebrae complex. SOV leaves the orbit through the superior orbital fissure. An important sign of pathology is dilation or thrombosis of SOV, which may occur in many orbital conditions and in carotid-cavernous sinus fistulas. AC is seen lateral to ICA. PCA is seen bilaterally, the terminal branches of BA. The inferior ophthalmic vein is not usually seen. Part of its course is demonstrated in Figure 2-24.

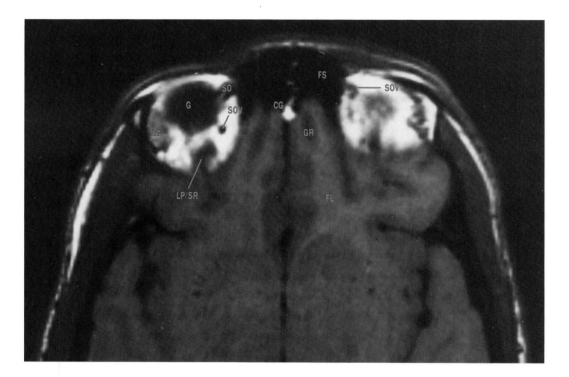

Figure 2-44 *T1-weighted, Superior Ophthalmic Vein* This image is identical to Figure 2-6. SOV extends from its origin at the angular vein into the orbit medially on the left side. On the right, SOV is seen in cross section. This section, combined with Figures 2-42 and 2-43, demonstrates the entire course of SOV from the angular vein to the superior orbital fissure.

CG	Crista Galli of Ethmoid Bone
FL	Frontal Lobe
FS	Frontal Sinus
G	Globe
GR	Gyrus Rectus of Frontal Lobe
LG	Lacrimal Gland
LP	Levator Palbebrae Superioris
SO	Superior Oblique Muscle
SOV	Superior Ophthalmic Vein
SR	Superior Rectus Muscle

ORBITAL FISSURES, CANALS, AND FORAMINA

2-3-1 CT: Axial, Contrast-Enhanced

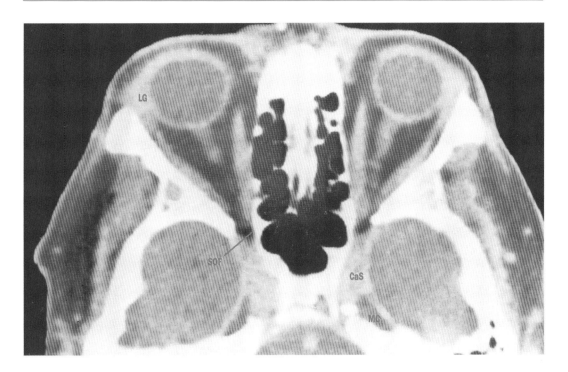

Figure 2-45 *Superior Orbital Fissure and Cavernous Sinus* In sections that contain the optic nerve, SOF may be confused with the optic foramen (see Figure 2-28). CaS is located lateral to the sphenoid sinus and the pituitary gland. Cranial nerves III, IV, V-1, and VI may be seen as lucencies within CaS, but are better seen on coronal sections (see Figure 6-8). MC contains the geniculate ganglion of the trigeminal nerve.

CaS	Cavernous Sinus
LG	Lacrimal Gland
MC	Meckel's Cave
SOF	Superior Orbital Fissure

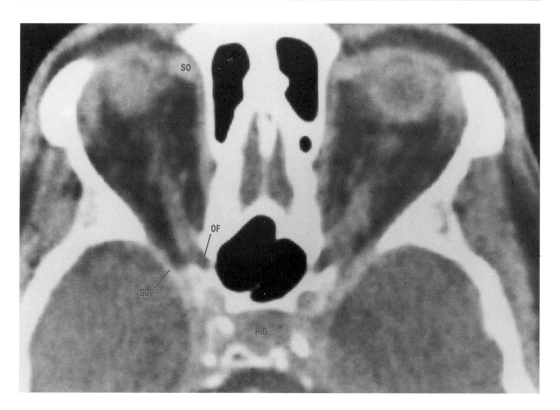

Figure 2-46 *Superior Orbital Fissure and Optic Foramen* At the apex of the orbit, SOF is seen separate from and lateral to OF. The paired SOF form a V-shape when viewed in the coronal plane, with the upper aspect of the V lateral to OF.

This slice is taken parallel to the orbitomeatal line; as a result, only the more superiorly located posterior part of OF is seen. (Figure 2-28 shows a slice through the entire OF.) Note the proximity of the optic nerves to PiG as the nerves enter the intracranial space, near the optic chiasm.

OF	Optic Foramen
PiG	Pituitary Gland
SO	Superior Oblique Muscle
SOF	Superior Orbital Fissure

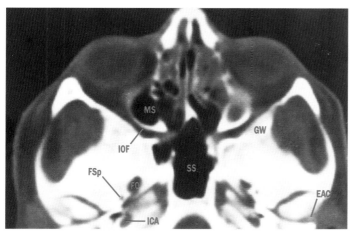

EAC	External Auditory Canal
FO	Foramen Ovale
FSp	Foramen Spinosum
GW	Greater Wing of Sphenoid Bone
ICA	Internal Carotid Artery
IOF	Inferior Orbital Fissure
MS	Maxillary Sinus
SS	Sphenoid Sinus

Figure 2-47 *Inferior Orbital Fissure* In this section, the posteromedial aspect of the orbital floor is replaced by the upper part of MS. FSp is posterolateral to FO. FO, which transmits the mandibular branch of the trigeminal nerve, is in the floor of the middle cranial fossa.

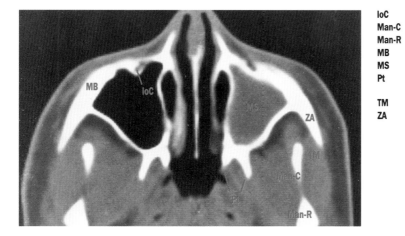

IoC	Infraorbital Canal
Man-C	Mandible—Coronoid Process
Man-R	Mandible—Ramus
MB	Maxillary Bone
MS	Maxillary Sinus
Pt	Pterygoid Plates of Sphenoid Bone
TM	Temporalis Muscle
ZA	Zygomatic Arch

Figure 2-48 *Infraorbital Canal* The lateral and medial Pt are separated by the pterygopalatine fossa. MS on the left is seen opacified. Note the location of IoC within the inferior orbital rim of MB. Orbital soft tissues or blood may fill MS after trauma or surgical decompression.

CHAPTER 3

Periorbital Structures

LACRIMAL SAC

3-1-1 MRI: Axial

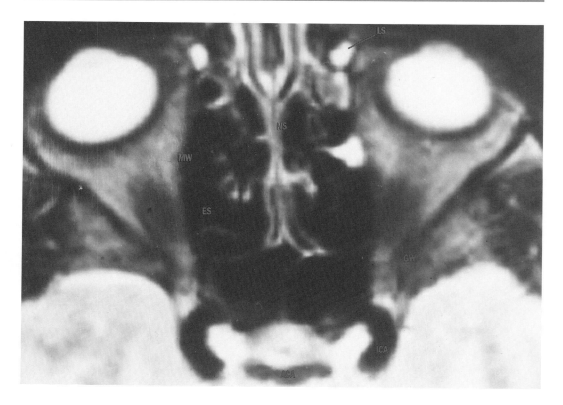

Figure 3-1 *T2-weighted, Lacrimal Sac* LS is clearly seen medial to the orbit bilaterally. LS enhances on T2-weighted scans because it is a water-filled structure enabling delineation from the adjacent air-filled spaces. GW forms the dark outline posteriorly on the lateral wall of the orbit. Because both bone and air are hypointense, the paper-thin bone of MW cannot be separated from the adjacent air-

filled ES. MW forms the lateral wall of ES. The appearance of bone on this scan should be compared with the CT in Figure 3-2, the level of which is slightly inferior to the plane of this image. CT is presently the preferred method for studying the bony course of the lacrimal drainage system. It is possible that MRI dacryocystography of the soft tissues may become technically feasible and clinically useful for some conditions.

ACA	Anterior Cerebral Artery
ES	Ethmoid Sinus
GW	Greater Wing of Sphenoid Bone
ICA	Internal Carotid Artery
LS	Lacrimal Sac
MW	Medial Wall of Orbit
NS	Nasal Septum

NASOLACRIMAL DUCT

3-2-1 CT: Axial, Bone Window

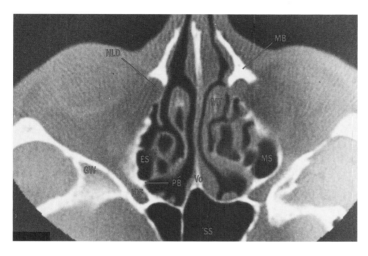

ES	Ethmoid Sinus
GW	Greater Wing of Sphenoid Bone
IOF	Inferior Orbital Fissure
MB	Maxillary Bone
MS	Maxillary Sinus
MT	Middle Turbinate
NLD	Nasolacrimal Duct
PB	Palatine Bone
SS	Sphenoid Sinus
Vo	Vomer

Figure 3-2 *Ethmoid and Maxillary Sinuses* NLD begins as a groove on the anterior lacrimal crest of MB. Surgical removal of bone from ES may injure NLD if back-biting forceps are used.

IOF lies between GW, MB, and the orbital process of PB, which contributes the posterior centimeter of the medial margin of IOF. PB may contain an air cell communicating with either the posterior ethmoid or sphenoid air cells.

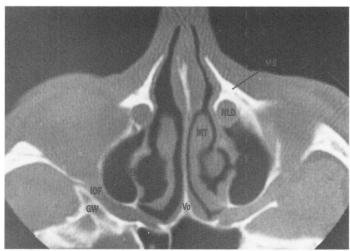

GW	Greater Wing of Sphenoid Bone
IOF	Inferior Orbital Fissure
MB	Maxillary Bone
MS	Maxillary Sinus
MT	Middle Turbinate
NLD	Nasolacrimal Duct
PB	Palatine Bone
Vo	Vomer

Figure 3-3 *Maxillary Sinus* Note that NLD has a closed outline at this level, inferior to the level in Figure 3-2. NLD opens into the inferior meatus of the nasal cavity, below the inferior turbinate. The anterior part of IOF lies between MB and GW.

PARANASAL (PERIORBITAL) SINUSES

3-3-1 CT: Axial, Bone Window

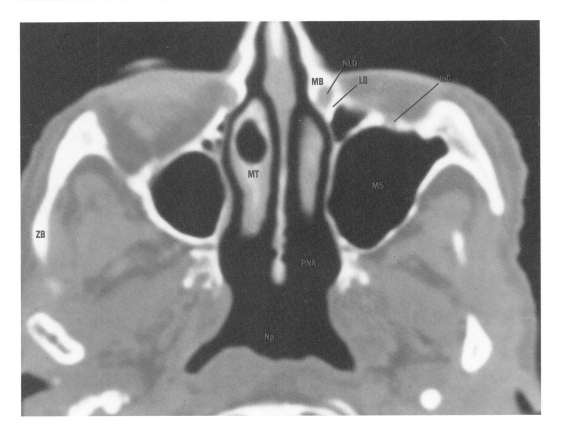

Figure 3-4 *Maxillary Sinus at Orbital Floor* The angulation of this section is more positive than that in Figure 3-3, although both contain the anterior orbital floor. NLD is medial to the inferior orbit and anterior to MT. A bulla is seen within MT. The presumed location of the descending process of LB is shown posteromedial to the bony nasolacrimal canal, while the lacrimal groove of MB comprises the remainder of its circumference. Tumors of Np at the fossa of Rosenmüller can invade the skull base and enter the inferior cavernous sinus, often leading to abducens nerve palsy and either pain or anesthesia of the lower face. This region is difficult to view without nasopharyngoscopy.

IoC	Infraorbital Canal
LB	Lacrimal Bone
MB	Maxillary Bone
MS	Maxillary Sinus
MT	Middle Turbinate
NLD	Nasolacrimal Duct
Np	Nasopharynx
PNA	Posterior Nasal Aperture
ZB	Zygomatic Bone

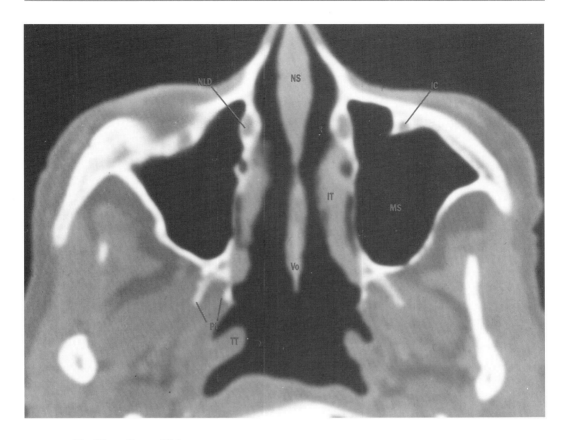

Figure 3-5 *Maxillary Sinus* This image is 6 mm inferior to Figure 3-4. NLD is seen passing lateral to the lateral edge of IT. TT is a cartilaginous process arising from the medial pterygoid plate that corresponds to the nasopharyngeal opening of the auditory (eustachian) tube (compare Figure 6-7).

IoC	Infraorbital Canal
IT	Inferior Turbinate
MS	Maxillary Sinus
NLD	Nasolacrimal Duct
NS	Nasal Septum
Pt	Pterygoid Plates of Sphenoid Bone (Medial and Lateral)
TT	Torus Tubarius
Vo	Vomer

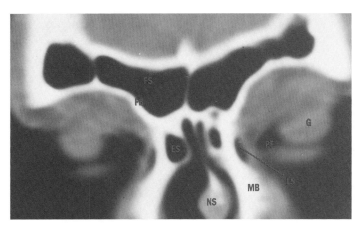

ES	Ethmoid Sinus
FB	Frontal Bone
FS	Frontal Sinus
G	Globe
LS	Lacrimal Sac
MB	Maxillary Bone
NS	Nasal Septum
PF	Palpebral Fissure

Figure 3-6 *Frontal Sinus* In this anterior slice, each LS can be seen medial to G. Note the deviation of NS. The frontal process of MB is medial to LS and forms the anterior lacrimal crest. ES can have bullae as far anterior as LS, as occurs here. Dacryocystorhinostomy must be carried through to the nasal cavity, so that intraoperative identification of an anterior ES bulla is imperative.

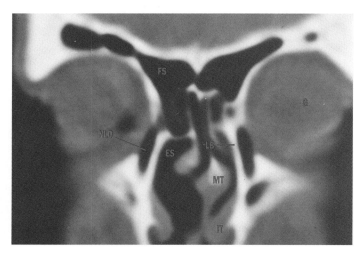

ES	Ethmoid Sinus
FS	Frontal Sinus
G	Globe
IT	Inferior Turbinate
LB	Lacrimal Bone
MT	Middle Turbinate
NLD	Nasolacrimal Duct

Figure 3-7 *Frontal and Ethmoid Sinuses* This slice is 4 mm posterior to Figure 3-6. The NLD descends through two bones: LB and the lacrimal process of IT (inferior concha). These two bones are relatively strong compared to the ethmoid bone. This is important during endoscopic sinus surgery because the bullae of ES are removed with back-biting forceps. The surgeon must detect the change in strength of the bone so as not to cut into bone surrounding NLD.

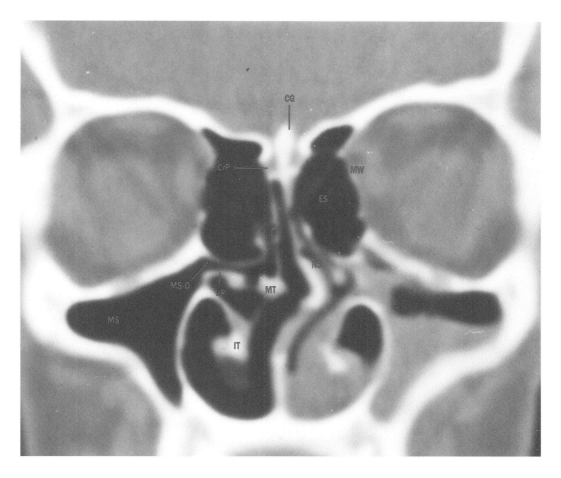

Figure 3-8 *Ostium of Maxillary Sinus* This slice is 6 mm posterior to Figure 3-7. MS-O is located rostrally and posteriorly on the medial wall of MS. It opens into the posterior part of the infundibulum of the middle meatus by passing under an ethmoidal bulla and over UP. Endoscopic sinus surgery begins by incising the lateral wall of the nose under MT (infundibulotomy), removing the bony UP, the anterior wall of the anterior bulla of ES, the basal lamina of MT, and finally the anterior wall of the sphenoid sinus. Injury to ocular structures can result from unplanned entry through MW into the orbit or the optic foramina. A medial orbital floor fracture or decompressive surgery for Graves' disease allows orbital contents to prolapse into MS-O and can cause obstructive sinus symptoms. NS is deviated to the patient's left, where it could interfere with sinus surgery.

CG	Crista Galli of Ethmoid Bone
CrP	Cribriform Plate of Ethmoid Bone
ES	Ethmoid Sinus
IT	Inferior Turbinate
MS	Maxillary Sinus
MS-O	Ostium of Maxillary Sinus
MT	Middle Turbinate
MW	Medial Wall of Orbit
NS	Nasal Septum
UP	Uncinate Process of Ethmoid Bone

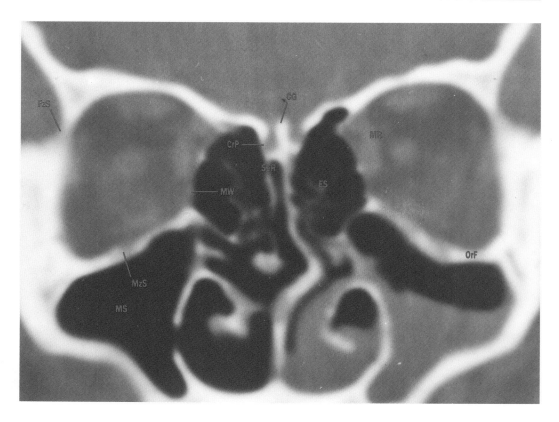

Figure 3-9 *Posterior Ethmoid Sinus* This section is 4 mm posterior to Figure 3-8. Note that OrF is seen in this CT with more detail and quality than is provided by the Waters view x-ray (Figure 2-39). The surgeon decompressing the medial orbit into ES should note that the top of MR can be below the level of CrP. Fracture of the medial wall of ES through CG can cause cerebrospinal fluid rhinorrea. The sphenoid sinus drains into SeR, the most posterior and rostral portion of the nasal cavity.

CG	Crista Galli of Ethmoid Bone
CrP	Cribriform Plate of Ethmoid Bone
ES	Ethmoid Sinus
FzS	Frontozygomatic Suture
MR	Medial Rectus Muscle
MS	Maxillary Sinus
MW	Medial Wall of Orbit
MzS	Maxillozygomatic Suture
OrF	Orbital Floor
SeR	Sphenoethmoidal Recess

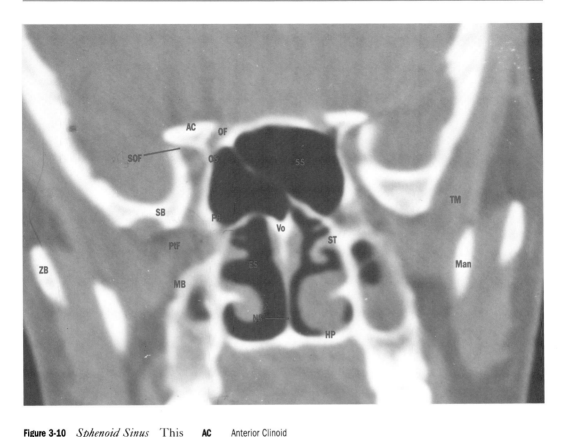

Figure 3-10 *Sphenoid Sinus* This slice is 24 mm posterior to Figure 3-9. The marrow cavity of AC can be seen in this bone window. This space may sometimes be aerated and be mistaken for OF on optic foramen views. The bony floor of OF is seen, but the roof is not because its posterior portion is composed of dura (the falciform fold). The orbital process of PB forms the medial aspect of the posterior inferior orbital fissure. The horizontal plates of PB constitute the posterior portion of HP, forming a ridge in the midline, the posterior nasal spine.

AC	Anterior Clinoid
ES	Ethmoid Sinus
HP	Hard Palate
Man	Mandible
MB	Maxillary Bone
NS	Nasal Septum
OF	Optic Foramen
OS	Optic Strut of Sphenoid Bone
PB	Palatine Bone
PtF	Pterygopalatine Fossa
SB	Sphenoid Bone
SOF	Superior Orbital Fissure
SS	Sphenoid Sinus
ST	Superior Turbinate
TM	Temporalis Muscle
Vo	Vomer
ZB	Zygomatic Bone

CANALS AND FORAMINA

3-4-1 CT: Coronal, Bone Window

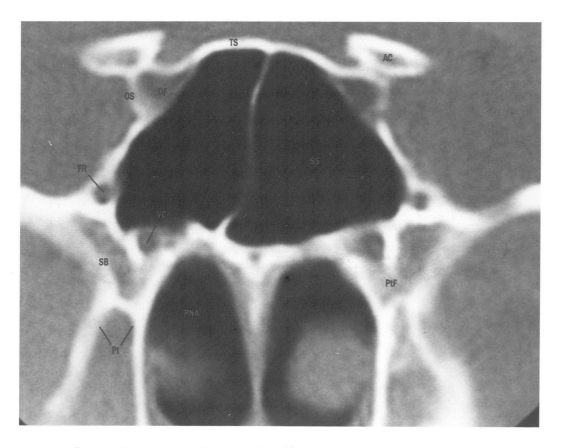

Figure 3-11 *Foramen Rotundum and Vidian Canal* FR lies between the lateral wall of SS and the root of the greater wing of the sphenoid bone. It contains the maxillary branch of the trigeminal nerve. VC is medial and inferior to FR. FR and VC are foramina in SB that open into PtF. Note that FR is lateral to VC; this relationship is analogous to the trigeminal nerve being lateral to the intracavernous internal carotid artery, the outer fascia of which conducts the sympathetic fibers, which join with the parasympathetic greater superficial petrosal nerve to become the vidian nerve (nerve of the pterygoid canal).

AC	Anterior Clinoid
FR	Foramen Rotundum
OF	Optic Foramen
OS	Optic Strut of Sphenoid Bone
PNA	Posterior Nasal Aperture
Pt	Pterygoid Plates of Sphenoid Bone
PtF	Pterygopalatine Fossa
SB	Sphenoid Bone
SS	Sphenoid Sinus
TS	Tuberculum Sella
VC	Vidian (Pterygoid) Canal

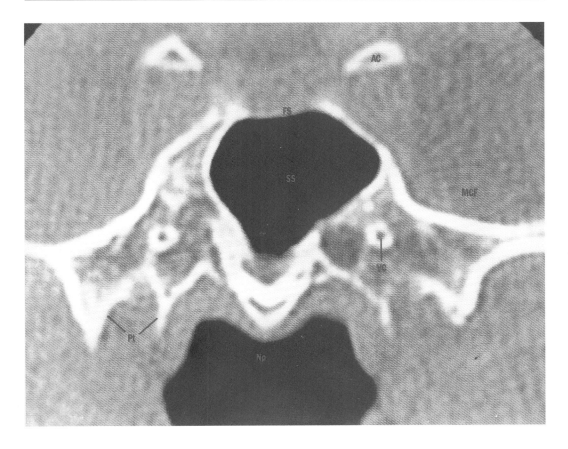

Figure 3-12 *Vidian Canal* This section is posterior to Figure 3-11. Because this is a bone-window image, the soft tissue outline of the cavernous sinus is barely detectable. VC extends forward with the foramen lacerum into the pterygopalatine fossa. It carries the vidian nerve, which supplies the parasympathetic innervation to the lacrimal gland from the greater superficial petrosal nerve, as well as sympathetic supply from the deep petrosal nerve.

AC	Anterior Clinoid
FS	Floor of Sella
MCF	Middle Cranial Fossa
Np	Nasopharynx
Pt	Pteryoid Plates of Sphenoid Bone
SS	Sphenoid Sinus
VC	Vidian (Pterygoid) Canal

CHAPTER 4

Brain

GENERAL

4-1-1 MRI: Axial

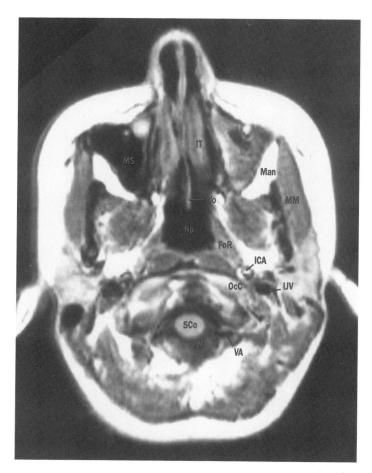

FM	Foramen Magnum
FoR	Fossa of Rosenmüller
ICA	Internal Carotid Artery
IJV	Internal Jugular Vein
IT	Inferior Turbinate
Man	Mandible
MM	Masseter Muscle
MS	Maxillary Sinus
Np	Nasopharynx
OcC	Occipital Condyle
SCo	Spinal Cord
VA	Vertebral Artery
Vo	Vomer

Figure 4-1 *T1-weighted, Foramen Magnum* Disorders in the region of FM may cause downbeat nystagmus. Congenital dilation of the spinal canal is known as *hydromyelia* and frequently coexists with Arnold-Chiari malformation and myelomeningocele. Syringomyelia is a cavitation of the cervical spinal cord. If the cavitation extends into the medulla oblongata, it is called *syringobulbia.* The two main types of Arnold-Chiari malformations are defined by their radiologic appearance. Type I presents with a low position of the cerebellar tonsils, which protrude through FM to reach the level of the arches of the first and second cervical vertebrae. There is effacement of FM, and the tonsils take on a peg-like appearance. Type I may either be asymptomatic or not become symptomatic until adulthood. Type II involves caudal displacement of the medulla, cerebellar vermis, and tonsils into the cervical spinal cord through a dilated FM. FoR is the location of posterior nasopharyngeal tumors, which can invade the inferior cavernous sinus and cause sixth-nerve palsies and pain or anesthesia in the distribution of the third division of the trigeminal nerve. Imaging studies are useful in the localization of tumors in this region, as they cannot be visualized directly. Endoscopic nasopharyngoscopy can be used to examine FoR.

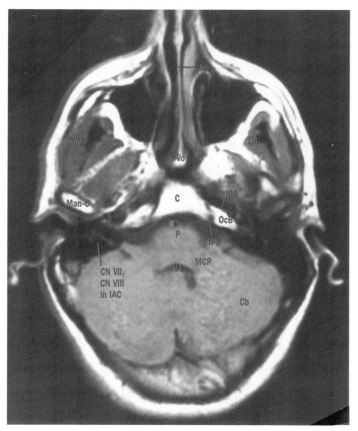

C	Clivus
Cb	Cerebellum
CN VII	Facial Nerve
CN VIII	Vestibulocochlear Nerve
IAC	Internal Auditory Canal
ICA	Internal Carotid Artery
IPS	Inferior Petrosal Sinus
Man-C	Coronoid Process of Mandible
MCP	Middle Cerebellar Peduncle
MM	Masseter Muscle
NS	Nasal Septum
OcB	Occipital Bone
P	Pons
TM	Temporalis Muscle
V4	Fourth Ventricle
Vo	Vomer

Figure 4-2 *T1-weighted, Cerebellar Hemispheres* The jugular tubercles of OcB lie lateral to C. They lie directly above the hypoglossal canal. Inferiorly, the jugular tubercles are grooved by IPS; posteriorly, they are grooved by the sigmoid sinuses at the point where they pass through the jugular foramen, becoming the internal jugular veins. CN VII and CN VIII are seen entering IAC. The midline structure in the nose consists of the cartilaginous NS anteriorly and the bony Vo posteriorly. ICA follows an oblique course anterior to OcB. Man-C is bordered internally by TM and externally by MM. A blood flow artifact from ICA extends in the anteroposterior direction in this and the next three figures. Here it extends through the left MCP.

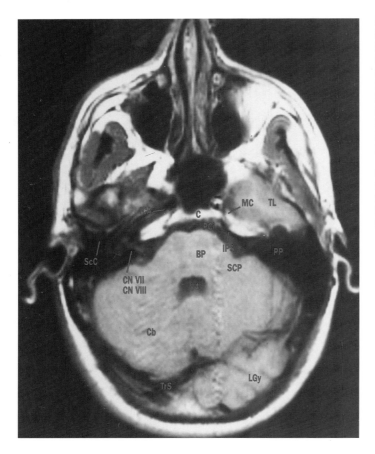

BP	Basis Pontis
C	Clivus
Cb	Cerebellum
CN VII	Facial Nerve
CN VIII	Vestibulocochlear Nerve
ICA	Internal Carotid Artery
IPS	Inferior Petrosal Sinus
LGy	Lingual Gyrus
MC	Meckel's Cave
PCi	Pontine Cistern
PP	Petrous Pyramid of Temporal Bone
ScC	Semicircular Canal
SCP	Superior Cerebellar Peduncle
TL	Temporal Lobe
TrS	Transverse Sinus
V4	Fourth Ventricle

Figure 4-3 *T1-weighted, Mid-Pons* C is a grooved region of bone that bridges the developmental spheno-occipital synchondrosis, lying in front of the foramen magnum inferiorly. Superiorly, C is continuous with the dorsum sellae and is seen as a midline structure anterior and inferior to the upper pons near the cerebral flexure. Irregularities in the floor of the middle cranial fossa, in the region of the squamous portion of the temporal bone, create the indented appearance at the posterior margin of the left TL.

SCP contains fibers coming from the dentate nucleus of Cb to the contralateral red nucleus of the midbrain. This forms one leg of Meynart's (myoclonic) triangle; the other two legs are the central tegmental tract (connecting the red nucleus to the ipsilateral inferior olivary nucleus) and the olivodental fibers connecting the inferior olivary nucleus and the contralateral dentate nucleus. Lesions within this anatomic loop produce various types of nystagmus, including oculopalatal myoclonus.

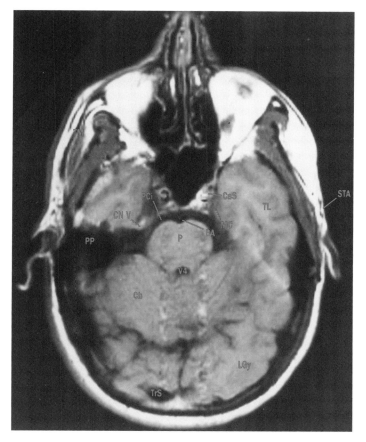

BA	Basilar Artery
CaS	Cavernous Sinus
Cb	Cerebellum
CN V	Trigeminal Nerve
LGy	Lingual Gyrus
MC	Meckel's Cave
P	Pons
PCi	Pontine Cistern
PP	Petrous Pyramid of Temporal Bone
STA	Superficial Temporal Artery
TL	Temporal Lobe
TM	Temporalis Muscle
TrS	Transverse Sinus
V4	Fourth Ventricle

Figure 4-4 *T1-weighted, Fourth Ventricle* The roof of V4 is formed in part by the anterior medullary velum, a thin lamina of white substance containing the decussation of the trochlear nerves. CN V can be seen in PCi, heading toward the Gasserian ganglion in MC. The inferior aspect of CaS is seen below the level of the pituitary gland. TrS is seen near its origin from the torcula. STA and veins are anterior to the auricle of the external ear, corresponding to the appoximate lower limit of incision for temporal artery biopsy. TM is covered by a fatty external fascia lateral to the orbit. LGy is the lowest portion of the occipital lobe and lies below the calcarine fissure. LGy and Cb are separated by the tentorium cerebelli, which is not seen because it is in the axial plane. TrS runs in the attached margin of the tentorium cerebelli. The fusiform or lateral occipitotemporal gyrus of TL extends forward into the anterior portion of the middle cranial fossa.

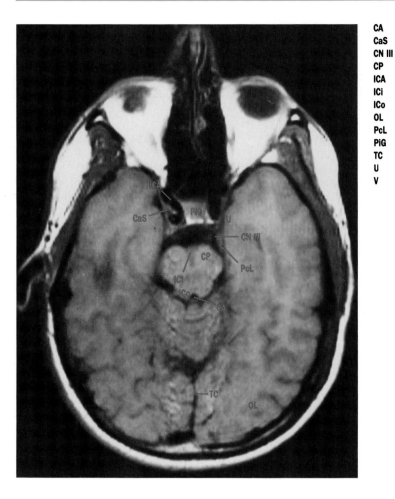

CA	Cerebral Aqueduct
CaS	Cavernous Sinus
CN III	Oculomotor Nerve
CP	Cerebral Peduncle
ICA	Internal Carotid Artery
ICi	Interpeduncular Cistern
ICo	Inferior Colliculus
OL	Occipital Lobe
PcL	Petroclinoid Ligament
PiG	Pituitary Gland
TC	Tentorium Cerebelli
U	Uncus of Temporal Lobe
V	Vermis of Cerebellum

Figure 4-5 *T1-weighted, Lower Midbrain* Fibers from ICo project to the ipsilateral medial geniculate body and are involved with auditory perception. The trochlear nerve nucleus is located in the peraqueductal gray matter of the midbrain at this level. CN III leaves CP as rootlets that become a single bundle within ICi and extend anteriorly to enter the superior aspect of CaS. CN III can be compressed by herniation of U through TC. The abducens nerve passes under PcL (Gruber's ligament) to enter CaS. The sixth nerve is tethered under PcL in Dorello's canal; this is where increased intracranial pressure causes sixth-nerve palsies. Note the flow void of ICA within CaS. This blood flow creates a noisy band of artifact in the anteroposterior direction that overlies V and the adjacent OL.

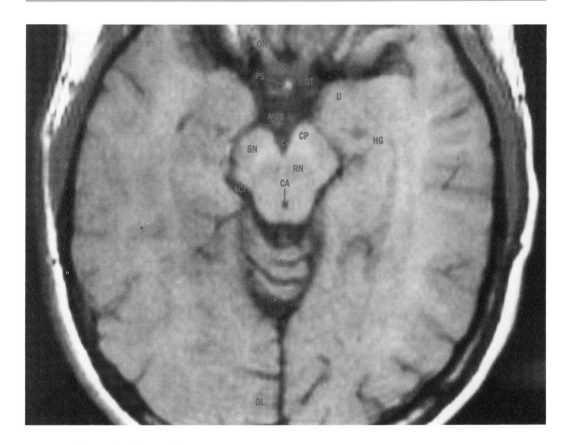

Figure 4-6 *T1-weighted, Cerebral Aqueduct* This section is at a level between the superior and inferior colliculi in the tectum of the midbrain and provides an excellent view of CA connecting the third and fourth ventricles. The intra-axial (intra–brain-stem) fibers of the oculomotor nerve course from their origin in this region through RN and CP. ACi is seen in its circummesencephalic location anterior to and continuous with the quadrigeminal plate cistern. MaB is a prominent structure between PS and the midbrain.

ACi	Ambient Cistern
CA	Cerebral Aqueduct
CP	Cerebral Peduncle
HG	Hippocampal Gyrus
ICi	Interpeduncular Cistern
MaB	Mamillary Body
OC	Optic Chiasm
OL	Occipital Lobe
ON	Optic Nerve
OT	Optic Tract
PS	Pituitary Stalk
RN	Red Nucleus
SN	Substantia Nigra
U	Uncus of Temporal Lobe
V	Vermis of Cerebellum

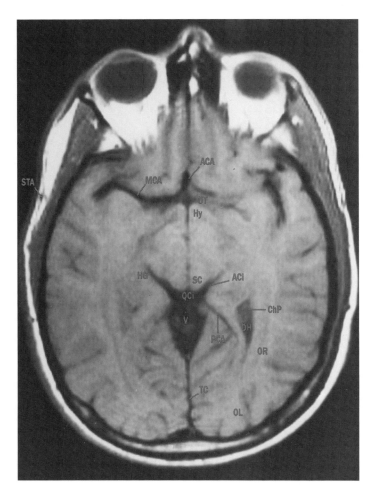

ACA	Anterior Cerebral Artery
ACi	Ambient Cistern
ChP	Choroid Plexus
HG	Hippocampal Gyrus
Hy	Hypothalamus
MCA	Middle Cerebral Artery
OH	Occipital Horn of Lateral Ventricle
OL	Occipital Lobe
OR	Optic Radiation
OT	Optic Tract
PCA	Posterior Cerebral Artery
QCi	Quadrigeminal Plate Cistern
SC	Superior Colliculus
STA	Superficial Temporal Artery
TC	Tentorium Cerebelli
V	Vermis of Cerebellum

Figure 4-7 *T1-weighted, Upper Midbrain* The plane of this section extends from SC posteriorly in the tectum of the midbrain through the tegmentum and OT anteriorly. The tectal and pretectal regions contain structures important for internal and external ocular movements. In addition, the afferent pupillary pathway courses through this region en route to the Edinger-Westphal nucleus. The oculomotor nerve nucleus is located in the dorsal midbrain at the level of SC. Upward herniation of V through the notch of TC may cause abnormalities of oculomotor function. The A1 segment of ACA arises from the bifurcation of the internal carotid artery in the interpeduncular cistern and runs above the optic nerve, where it is seen in longitudinal section at the approximate level of the anterior communicating artery. The artery then turns vertically as the A2 segment of ACA and runs upward around the genu of the corpus callosum. Both the A1 and the A2 segments are seen in this 6-mm slice.

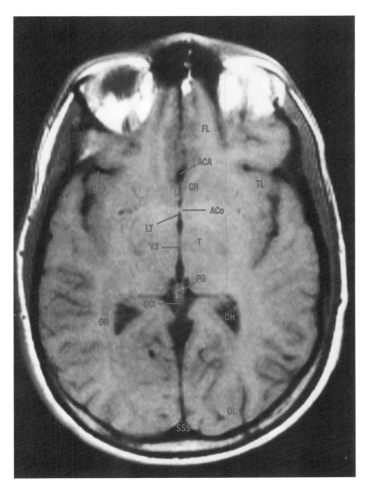

ACA	Anterior Cerebral Artery
ACo	Anterior Commisure
CN	Caudate Nucleus
FL	Frontal Lobe
LCF	Lateral Cerebral Fissure
LT	Lamina Terminalis
OH	Occipital Horn of Lateral Ventricle
OL	Occipital Lobe
OR	Optic Radiation
PG	Pineal Gland
QCi	Quadrigeminal Plate Cistern
SSS	Superior Sagittal Sinus
T	Thalamus
TL	Temporal Lobe
V3	Third Ventricle

Figure 4-8 *T1-weighted, Third Ventricle* LT is the anterior boundary of V3 and is the cranial end of the primitive neural tube. Abnormalities of LT are associated with septo-optic dysplasia. ACo is directly anterior to LT. PG is seen within QCi, which is continuous with the superior cerebellar cistern. OR is located within the external sagittal stratum of the internal capsule. The region just lateral to the tip of the front leader for OR is designated as the *temporal isthmus*. It contains white matter tracts relating to sensation of the opposite extremities and motor control of the opposite leg. A stroke involving the anterior choroidal artery can injure the temporal isthmus, causing contralateral hemianopia, hemisensory defects, and hemiplegia. Dominant hemisphere lesions can also produce aphasia, while nondominant hemisphere symptoms include autopagnosia (somatotopagnosia), wherein the patient does not recognize portions of his own body nor the body parts of other people.

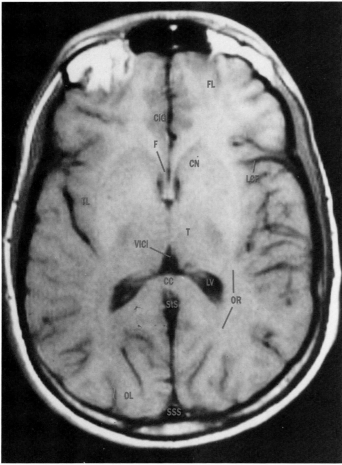

CiG	Cingulate Gyrus
CC	Corpus Callosum
CN	Caudate Nucleus
F	Fornix
FL	Frontal Lobe
LCF	Lateral Cerebral Fissure
LV	Lateral Ventricle
OL	Occipital Lobe
OR	Optic Radiation
SSS	Superior Sagittal Sinus
StS	Straight Sinus
T	Thalamus
TL	Temporal Lobe
VICi	Cistern of Velum Interpositum

Figure 4-9 *T1-weighted, Cistern of Velum Interpositum* VICi is the triangular structure in the plane between the temporal horns of each LV. VICi is an anterosuperior extension of the quadrigeminal plate cistern. It lies above the suprapineal recess of the third ventricle. The columns of F meet in the anterior third ventricle. StS lies immediately behind the splenium of CC. LCF separates FL from TL. The calcarine cortex of OL is labeled. The portion of OL superior to the calcarine fissure is the cuneus; the portion inferior to the fissure is the lingual gyrus. The division can be appreciated in coronal and sagittal sections (see Figures 4-33 and 4-38), but not on axial sections, where the fissure is parallel to the plane of imaging. T lies medial to the posterior limb of the internal capsule.

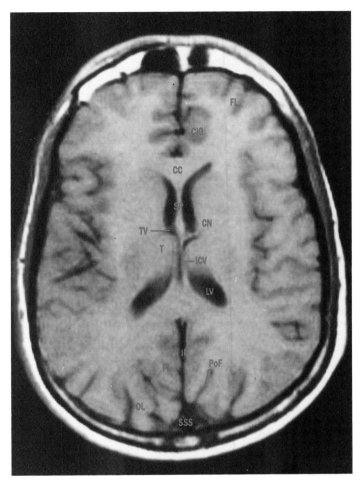

CC	Corpus Callosum
CiG	Cingulate Gyrus
CN	Caudate Nucleus
FL	Frontal Lobe
ICV	Internal Cerebral Vein
IF	Interhemispheric Fissure
LV	Lateral Ventricle
OL	Occipital Lobe
PL	Parietal Lobe
PoF	Parieto-occipital Fissure
SP	Septum Pellucidum
SSS	Superior Sagittal Sinus
T	Thalamus
TV	Thalamostriate Vein

Figure 4-10 *T1-weighted, Genu of Corpus Callosum* The head of CN indents the lateral aspect of LV. The frontal horn extends anteriorly from the body of LV, while the trigone runs posteriorly. SP separates the two LV. The rostrum and splenium of CC are seen anteriorly and posteriorly, respectively. ICV is a paired midline structure located in the roof of the third ventricle formed by the merger of TV and choroidal veins below the foramen of Monro. TV is situated between CN and T. Posteriorly, below the splenium of CC, both ICV join to form the vein of Galen (the great cerebral vein).

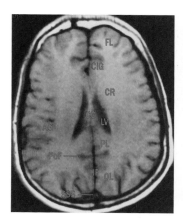 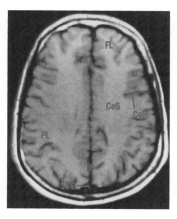 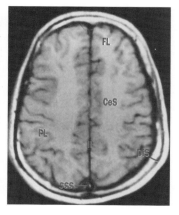

Figure 4-11 *T1-weighted, Body of Lateral Ventricle* The body of CC is located between the bodies of each LV. In some individuals, the body of LV may be superior to the body of CC. IF separates FL and PL and is seen anterior and posterior to LV. The cuneus of OL can be identified as the region of OL posterior to PoF.

AG	Angular Gyrus
CC	Corpus Callosum
CiG	Cingulate Gyrus
CR	Corona Radiata
FL	Frontal Lobe
IF	Interhemispheric Fissure
LV	Lateral Ventricle
OL	Occipital Lobe
PL	Parietal Lobe
PoF	Parieto-occipital Fissure
SSS	Superior Sagittal Sinus

Figure 4-12 *T1-weighted, Parietal Lobe Above Corpus Callosum* The precuneus of PL is superior and anterior to the cuneus of the occipital lobe. A common misconception is that sections at this or higher levels contain the occipital lobe. Lesions of CeS and PL at this level may be associated with homonymous inferior quadrantic visual field defects or abnormal optokinetic nystagmus. SSS is seen posteriorly within IF.

CeF	Central Fissure
CeS	Centrum Semiovale
CiG	Cingulate Gyrus
FL	Frontal Lobe
IF	Interhemispheric Fissure
PL	Parietal Lobe
SSS	Superior Sagittal Sinus

Figure 4-13 *T1-weighted, Centrum Semiovale* FL is labeled in the middle frontal gyrus, which contains the frontal motor eye field (area 8 of Brodmann). The low intensity within IF corresponds to the falx cerebri. SSS can be seen at both the anterior and the posterior aspects of IF.

CeS	Centrum Semiovale
DiS	Diploic Space
FL	Frontal Lobe
IF	Interhemispheric Fissure
PL	Parietal Lobe
SSS	Superior Sagittal Sinus

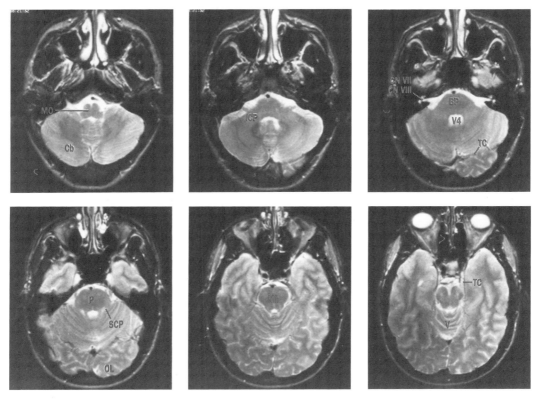

Figure 4-14 *T2-weighted, Lowest 6 Sections* This figure, along with Figures 4-15 and 4-16, displays images obtained on routine T2-weighted brain scans extending from the upper medulla through the parietal cortex, obtained at a slice thickness of 5 mm. These 18 slices contain the region of most interest in the evaluation of neuro-ophthalmic disorders. T2-weighted images are commonly used in the identification of pathologic conditions involving intracranial structures. The hallmark of a T2-weighted image is the intense appearance of structures with a high water content, including the cerebrospinal fluid, vitreous, and nasal mucosa. As a result, edema will often highlight an abnormal region due to a high signal of water. These sections can be evaluated for the anatomy of the normal soft tissue structures and the fluid-filled spaces. These multiple sections are presented to demonstrate the images comprising an entire brain scan and must be integrated in the routine of examining films in addition to looking for particular structures that are suspected locations of disease in the individual patient.

BP	Basis Pontis
Cb	Cerebellum
CN VII	Facial Nerve
CN VIII	Vestibulocochlear Nerve
ICP	Inferior Cerebellar Peduncle
Mb	Midbrain
MO	Medulla Oblongata
OL	Occipital Lobe
P	Pons
SCP	Superior Cerebellar Peduncle
TC	Tentorium Cerebelli
V	Vermis of Cerebellum
V4	Fourth Ventricle

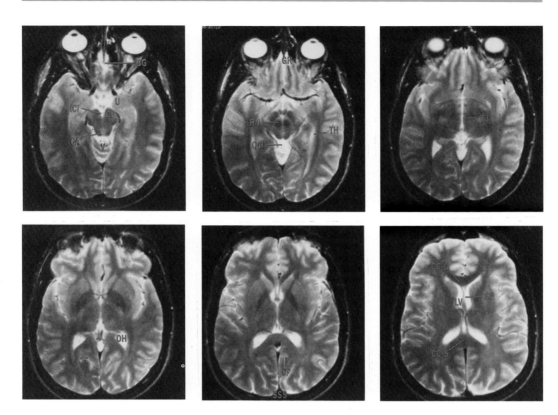

Figure 4-15 *T2-weighted, Middle 6 Sections* Review of serial slices enables following the course of the ventricular system upward from CA through V3 to LV. Noncommunicating hydrocephalus can occur due to obstruction of V4, CA, or V3. Downward herniation of U can cause oculomotor paralysis, and upward herniation of V can impair pupillary function and control of gaze. Notice that on T2-weighted scans, the gray matter appears lighter than the white matter. This is opposite to the pattern seen on T1-weighted scans (see Figure 4-6). On proton-density-weighted images, gray and white matter appear similar to each other (see Table 1-1).

CA	Cerebral Aqueduct
CC-G	Corpus Callosum—Genu
CC-S	Corpus Callosum—Splenium
CF	Calcarine Fissure
CG	Crista Galli of Ethmoid Bone
CP	Cerebral Peduncle
GR	Gyrus Rectus of Frontal Lobe
ICi	Interpeduncular Cistern
LV	Lateral Ventricle
OH	Occipital Horn of Lateral Ventricle
QCi	Quadrigeminal Plate Cistern
RN	Red Nucleus
SP	Septum Pellucidum
SSS	Superior Sagittal Sinus
TH	Temporal Horn of Lateral Ventricle
U	Uncus of Temporal Lobe
V	Vermis of Cerebellum
V3	Third Ventricle

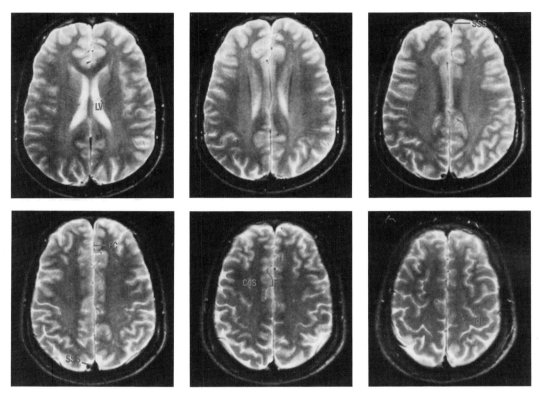

Figure 4-16 *T2-weighted, Highest 6 Sections* These sections through the cerebral hemispheres should be inspected for evidence of asymmetry, particularly midline shift. The cerebral sulci are regions of the subarachnoid space interspersed between the gyri of the cerebral lobes. Prominence of the sulci is generally a sign of cerebral atrophy, whereas loss of this prominence is seen in cases of brain edema. Abnormal anatomic patterns occur as a result of developmental abnormalities. CeS is an area containing projection fibers from the corticospinal tract, the corpus callosum, and between cortical association regions. The name CeS is derived from the semioval shape of the white matter deep to the surface cortex in sections above the level of the corpus callosum. It is important to realize that the upper cuts do not contain the occipital lobes.

CeS	Centrum Semiovale
FC	Falx Cerebri
FL	Frontal Lobe
IF	Interhemispheric Fissure
LV	Lateral Ventricle
PL	Parietal Lobe
SSS	Superior Sagittal Sinus

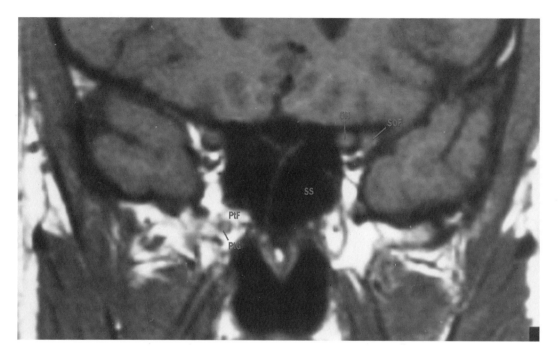

Figure 4-17 *T1-weighted, Optic Foramen and Superior Orbital Fissure* This is the first in a series of 9 T1-weighted coronal images taken at a thickness of 3 mm. This section is 3 mm posterior to Figure 2-15. T1-weighted images are often used in evaluating intracranial lesions in the anterior visual pathway because they provide better anatomic definition of small structures than is provided by T2-weighted images, which are the standard imaging technique for most intracranial pathology. ON is seen in the optic foramen, which is located medial to SOF. These two structures are separated by the optic strut of the sphenoid bone. The individual cranial nerves within SOF cannot be distinguished.

ON	Optic Nerve
PtF	Pterygopalatine Fossa
PtG	Pterygopalatine Ganglion
SOF	Superior Orbital Fissure
SS	Sphenoid Sinus

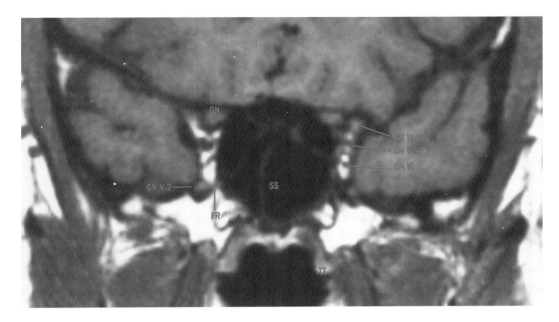

Figure 4-18 *T1-weighted, Optic Foramen and Anterior Cavernous Sinus* The intracavernous course of CN III, IV, V, and VI is distinguished more clearly on MRI than CT (compare Figure 6-8). CN IV is inferolateral to CN III, but cannot be delineated because of its small size, only 3400 axons. CN V-1 lies below CN III. CN V-1 divides into three branches in the most anterior part of the cavernous sinus, the largest of which is the frontal nerve. CN V-2 has already departed from the cavernous sinus and is seen as a separate structure below the cavernous sinus, in FR. The nerves cannot be labeled with certainty because of their shifting relationships within the cavernous sinus. Note the superomedial course of ON as it passes from the orbit into the brain. At this level, it is difficult to be certain whether all borders of ON are within the optic foramen, in which case ON is separated from the cavernous sinus contents by the optic strut of the sphenoid bone. Posterior to the point where the inferior border of ON exits the optic foramen, the superior border is covered by a layer of dura, the falciform fold. On T1-weighted scans, the sphenoid bone, air in SS, and dura forming the falciform fold overlying the nerve all have a similar appearance. TT (or tubal elevation) is comprised of cartilage arising from the medial pterygoid process; it marks the nasopharyngeal opening of the auditory (eustachian) tube.

CN III	Oculomotor Nerve
CN V-1	Trigeminal Nerve—1st Division
CN V-2	Trigeminal Nerve—2nd Division
CN VI	Abducens Nerve
FR	Foramen Rotundum
ON	Optic Nerve
SS	Sphenoid Sinus
TT	Torus Tubarius

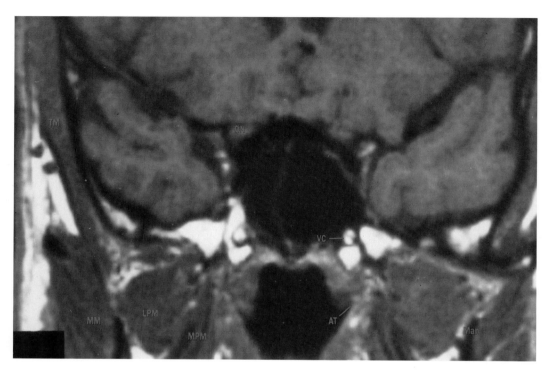

Figure 4-19 *T1-weighted, Intracranial Optic Nerve* ON at this level is medial to the internal carotid artery as it rises and approaches the optic chiasm (see Figure 4-20). VC transmits the vidian nerve branches of CN VII en route to the pterygopalatine ganglion (Figure 2-24), where they synapse and pass via the zygomaticotemporal branch of CN V-2 to the lacrimal nerve of CN V-1. The vidian nerve includes sympathetic nerves that leave the superior portion of the ca- rotid canal as the deep petrosal nerve and fibers originating in the lacrimal and superior salivary nuclei that exit the brain as a part of CN VII and con- tinue from the temporal bone as the greater superficial petro- sal nerve. Dysfunction of ON immediately anterior to the chiasm gives rise to a supero- temporal visual field defect on the opposite side because of involvement of the inferonasal retinal crossing fibers in Wil- brand's knee. This field de- fect, combined with a central scotoma on the side of the le- sion involving ON, is called a *junctional scotoma.*

AT	Auditory Tube
LPM	Lateral Pterygoid Muscle
Man	Mandible
MM	Masseter Muscle
MPM	Medial Pterygoid Muscle
ON	Optic Nerve
TM	Temporalis Muscle
VC	Vidian Canal

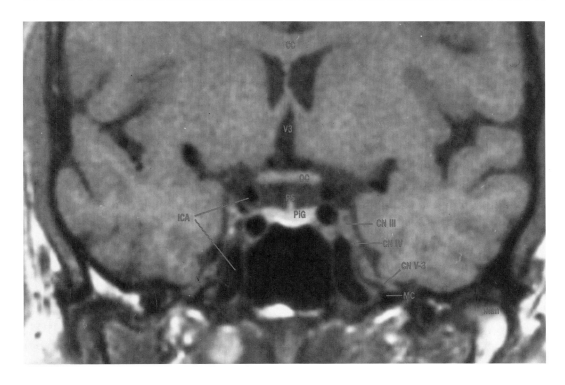

Figure 4-20 *T1-weighted, Optic Chiasm and Anterior Pituitary Gland* The intracavernous ICA is seen both in longitudinal and in cross sections because of its S-shaped course (compare with the sagittal view, Figure 2-24). ICA is also seen in the suprasellar cistern, inferolateral to OC. CN V-3 is seen as it exits MC and passes into the foramen ovale (compare with the CT in Figure 2-47). The supraoptic recess of V3 is seen above OC. Bitemporal hemianopia is the hall-mark of chiasmal dysfunction. If compression of OC comes from below, the field defect begins superiorly and progresses in a clockwise direction in the right visual field and in a counterclockwise direction in the left. PiG lies approximately 10 mm below the chiasm. Before visual field defects become apparent, pituitary adenomas must be large enough to break through the diaphragma sellae and extend into the suprasellar cistern, where they compress the visual pathway. If OC is compressed from above, as in a craniopharyngioma, the inferior temporal fields may be the first affected.

CC	Corpus Callosum
CN III	Oculomotor Nerve
CN IV	Trochlear Nerve
CN V-3	Trigeminal Nerve—3rd Division
ICA	Internal Carotid Artery
Man	Mandible
MC	Meckel's Cave
OC	Optic Chiasm
PiG	Pituitary Gland
PS	Pituitary Stalk
V3	Third Ventricle

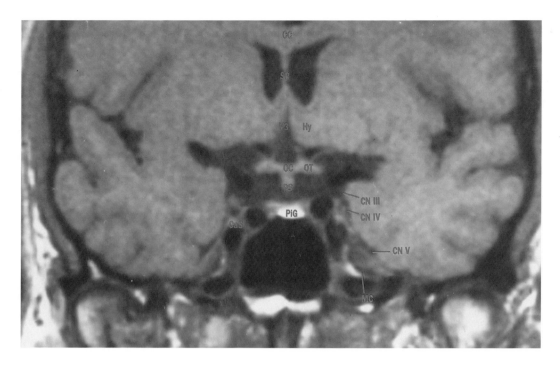

Figure 4-21 *T1-weighted, Optic Chiasm at Junction With Optic Tracts* The origin of each OT is seen arising from OC. OC is bounded above by the supra-optic recess of V3 and below by PS, which connects Hy to PiG. MC is an invagination of dura mater along the petrous portion of the temporal bone, beneath the superior petrosal sinus, which contains the gas-serian ganglion of CN V. The medial wall of MC fuses with the roof of CaS. SP divides the paired lateral ventricles. Its absence is a feature of de-Morsier's syndrome, with hypoplasia of the optic nerves and hypopituitarism. The supraoptic nucleus is located in the anterior Hy over the lateral border of OT. It receives ipsilateral and contralateral retino-hypothalamic projections and is concerned with the regulation of circadian rhythms.

CaS	Cavernous Sinus
CC	Corpus Callosum
CN III	Oculomotor Nerve
CN IV	Trochlear Nerve
CN V	Trigeminal Nerve
Hy	Hypothalamus
MC	Meckel's Cave
OC	Optic Chiasm
OT	Optic Tract
PiG	Pituitary Gland
PS	Pituitary Stalk
SP	Septum Pellucidum
V3	Third Ventricle

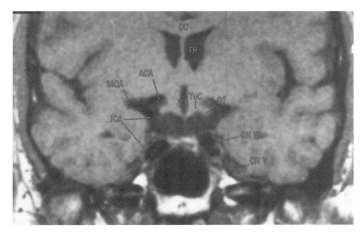

ACA	Anterior Cerebral Artery
CC	Corpus Callosum
CN III	Oculomotor Nerve
CN V	Trigeminal Nerve
FH	Frontal Horn of Lateral Ventricle
ICA	Internal Carotid Artery
MCA	Middle Cerebral Artery
OT	Optic Tract
TuC	Tuber Cinereum of Hypothalamus
V3	Third Ventricle

Figure 4-22 *T1-weighted, Anterior Optic Tract* Each OT is seen as a separate structure, poste-rior to the optic chiasm. Tu-mors involving TuC can cause hormonal dysfunctions, includ-ing precocious puberty. CN III passes through the subarach-noid space prior to penetrating the dura to enter the cavernous sinus. ACA and MCA can be seen as flow voids superior to the suprasellar portion of ICA.

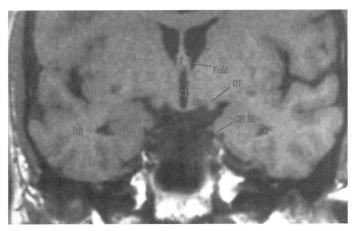

CN III	Oculomotor Nerve
F	Fornix
FoM	Foramen of Monro
Hy	Hypothalamus
OR	Optic Radiation
OT	Optic Tract
TH	Temporal Horn of Lateral Ventricle
U	Uncus of Temporal Lobe
V3	Third Ventricle

Figure 4-23 *T1-weighted, Optic Tract* OT is more lateral than in Figure 4-22 as it approaches the lateral geniculate body. Note the relationship of U to CN III. Herniation of the tem-poral lobe at this location may give rise to a dilated pupil (Hutchinson's pupil). This is the most anterior image con-taining TH. Following their exit from the lateral geniculate body, the inferior bundles of OR pass through the external sagittal stratum laterally and anteriorly and loop (Meyer's loop) around the tip of TH, where they turn posteriorly. The most anterior extent oc-curs at a point less than 1 cm lateral to the tip of TH. This is about 5 cm posterior to the tip of the temporal lobe. Ante-rior lesions of OT may result in noncongruous hemianopias because corresponding fibers from the two optic nerves do not occupy identical positions within OT at this location.

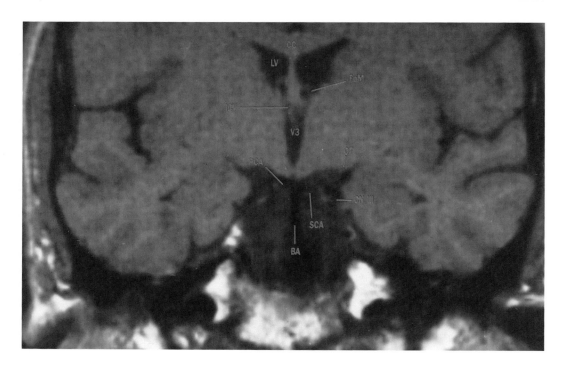

Figure 4-24 *T1-weighted, Posterior Optic Tract* BA is a midline structure anterior to the brain stem. Prior to its termination, it gives off SCA, while at its tip it bifurcates into the posterior cerebral arteries (PCA). CN III is seen passing between these vessels after multiple rootlets have consolidated into a single nerve anterior to the brain stem. Lesions involving OT may produce both an ipsilateral hemianopia and a contralateral relative afferent pupillary defect, the optic tract syndrome. This is because fibers from OT project to both the lateral geniculate body and the pretectal and suprachiasmatic nuclei. Involvement of OT prior to separation of the pupillary fibers in the region of the superior colliculus will produce a contralateral relative afferent pupillary defect. ICV is shown at its origin below FoM and the genu of CC (see Figure 4-10).

BA	Basilar Artery
CC	Corpus Callosum
CN III	Oculomotor Nerve
FoM	Foramen of Monro
ICV	Internal Cerebral Vein
LV	Lateral Ventricle
OT	Optic Tract
PCA	Posterior Cerebral Artery
SCA	Superior Cerebellar Artery
V3	Third Ventricle

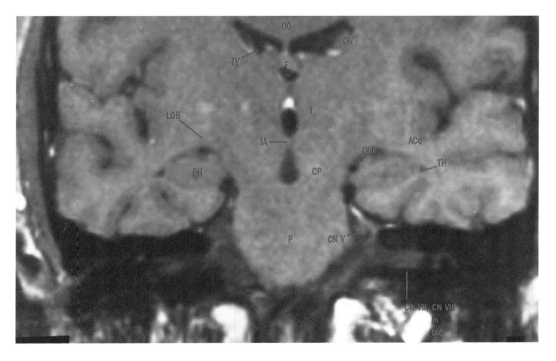

Figure 4-25 *T1-weighted, Lateral Geniculate Body* Compare this slice to Figures 4-29 and 5-14, T2-weighted images taken at the same level. The optic tract passes lateral to CP within the crural cistern to reach LGB. Note the relationship of the cerebrospinal-fluid–containing crural cistern, ChF, and TH. Although the latter two structures appear to be continuous, they are separated by a thin membrane composed of pia mater on one side and ependyma on the other. The teg-

mentum of the brain stem is seen extending downward to P. CC connects the cerebral hemispheres and may be absent in developmental abnormalities such as Aicardi's syndrome. The lateral portion of ACo provides interhemispheric connections for the temporal and frontal lobes. CN V is seen passing backward from the gasserian ganglion, approaching the lateral border of P. CN VII and VIII are seen leaving the lower border of P through the lateral pontine cistern into IAC. TV can be seen at the lateral margin of the lateral ventricle, separating CN from T.

ACo	Anterior Commissure
CC	Corpus Callosum
ChF	Choroidal Fissure
CN	Caudate Nucleus
CN V	Trigeminal Nerve
CN VII	Facial Nerve
CN VIII	Vestibulocochlear Nerve
CP	Cerebral Peduncle
F	Fornix
IA	Interthalamic Adhesion
IAC	Internal Auditory Canal
LGB	Lateral Geniculate Body
P	Pons
PH	Pes Hippocampus
T	Thalamus
TH	Temporal Horn of Lateral Ventricle
TV	Thalamostriate Vein

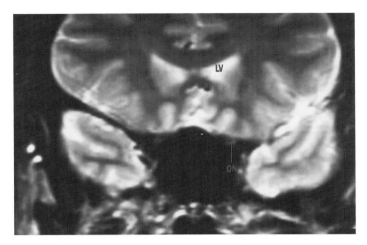

LV   Lateral Ventricle
ON Optic Nerve

terest are generally large; (2) the hyperintense appearance of the cerebrospinal fluid in the ventricular system aids in detecting displacement; and (3) pathologic processes are more easily detected on T2-weighted images than on T1-weighted images. However, the increased signal in the ventricles and cisterns obscures detail of fine structures. Compare the T1-weighted image of this same section, Figure 4-19. While the cerebrospinal fluid in LV becomes hyperintense in T2-weighted images, air and bone remain hypointense, as in T1-weighted images.

Figure 4-26 *T2-weighted, Intracranial Optic Nerve* This is the first of 10 T2-weighted sections of the afferent visual pathway, extending from the intracranial ON posteriorly to the occipital pole. T2-weighted images are frequently used to image the brain because (1) the structures of interest are generally large; (2)

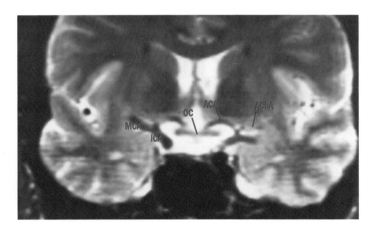

ACA   Anterior Cerebral Artery
AChA Anterior Choroidal Artery
ICA   Internal Carotid Artery
MCA Middle Cerebral Artery
OC   Optic Chiasm

hyperintensity of the chiasmatic cistern outside the vessels and the flow void within. As a result, the bifurcation of ICA into ACA and MCA is clearly seen. AChA, usually the final branch of the suprasellar ICA before the bifurcation, courses laterally into the crural cistern (a lateral extension of the chiasmatic cistern between the cerebral peduncle and the temporal lobe), where it supplies the optic tract.

Figure 4-27 *T2-weighted, Optic Chiasm* This image should be compared to the T1-weighted Figure 4-20, taken at the same level. Note the increased detail of sellar and cavernous sinus anatomy with T1 weighting. In contrast, the vascular structures are seen more clearly with T2 weighting due to the contrast between the

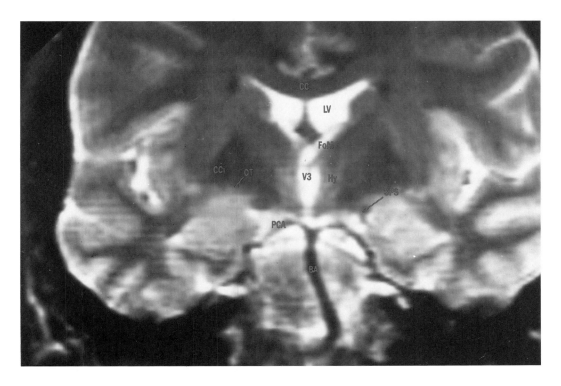

Figure 4-28 *T2-weighted, Optic Tract* OT is seen passing through CCi, lateral to Hy. FoM is not usually well seen unless there is cerebral atrophy, but can be identified by virtue of the intensity of the cerebrospinal fluid seen passing through FoM. Tumors associated with tuberous sclerosis may obstruct FoM, resulting in hydrocephalus and papilledema. The course of BA and its terminal branches, the posterior cerebral arteries (PCA),

are clearly seen (compare to the T1-weighted image at the same level, Figure 4-21). This section is just behind the posterior clinoid processes, where the tentorium cerebelli (not clearly seen) has its anterior attachment. However, the location of the tentorium can be assumed by the flow void created by SPS, which runs within its medial margin. The location of CN III, the oculomotor nerve, can be assumed to be within the hyperintense cerebrospinal fluid present just below SPS.

BA	Basilar Artery
CC	Corpus Callosum
CCi	Crural Cistern
FoM	Foramen of Monro
Hy	Hypothalamus
LV	Lateral Ventricle
OT	Optic Tract
PCA	Posterior Cerebral Artery
SPS	Superior Petrosal Sinus
V3	Third Ventricle

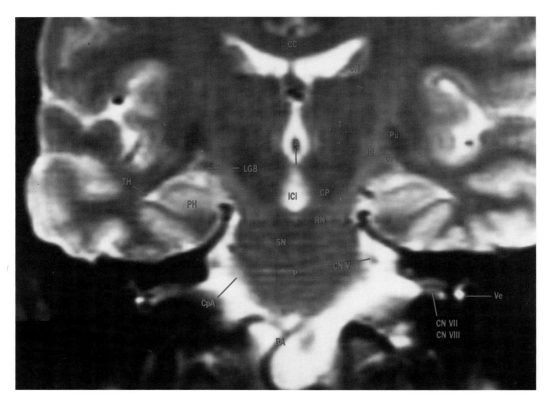

Figure 4-29 *T2-weighted, Lateral Geniculate Body* LGB is discussed in more detail in association with Figure 5-14. This image is at the same level as the T1-weighted Figure 4-25. BA is seen in front of P and is not usually straight or exactly midlline. The intra-axial course of CN III, the oculomotor nerve, passes through mesencephalic structures (including RN) en route to ICi. Lesions of CN III and RN produce Benedikt's syndrome, while lesions of CN III and the cerebral peduncles produce Weber's syndrome. CN VII and VIII pass through the lateral pontine cistern en route to the internal auditory canal. Their apparent division in the canal is an artifact due to the hypointense signal of the internal auditory artery. CC agenesis is a feature of developmental abnormalities such as Aicardi's syndrome. Iron deposition within GP may be seen in Hallervorden-Spatz syndrome. Lesions of the basal ganglia, including CN, GP, Pu, RN, and SN, give rise to extrapyramidal disorders; eg, blepharospasm, parkinsonism, dystonia, Wilson's disease, and Huntington's chorea. CP is shown in continuity with the posterior limb of IC.

BA	Basilar Artery
CC	Corpus Callosum
CN	Caudate Nucleus
CN V	Trigeminal Nerve
CN VII	Facial Nerve
CN VIII	Vestibulocochlear Nerve
CP	Cerebral Peduncle
CpA	Cerebellopontine Angle
GP	Globus Pallidus
IA	Interthalamic Adhesion
IC	Internal Capsule
ICi	Interpeduncular Cistern
LGB	Lateral Geniculate Body
P	Pons
PH	Pes Hippocampus
Pu	Putamen
RN	Red Nucleus
SN	Substantia Nigra
T	Thalamus
TH	Temporal Horn of Lateral Ventricle
Ve	Vestibule

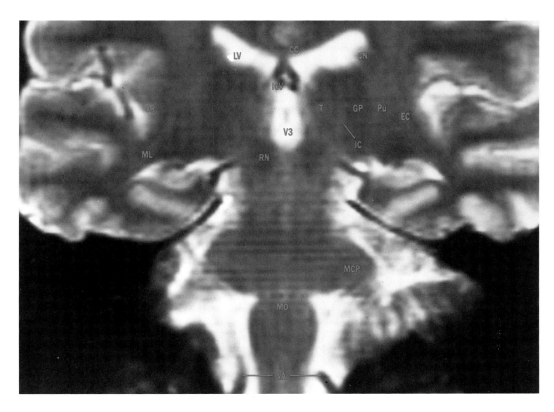

Figure 4-30 *T2-weighted, Thalamus, Posterior to Lateral Geniculate Body* At this level, T comprises the main gray matter structure on either side of V3. It is composed of medial, lateral, and ventral nuclei that cannot be distinguished. ICV are paired midline structures located in the roof of V3. The head of CN indents the infero- lateral aspect of LV. OR has reached a position lateral to LV. The dorsal bundles of OR are in the posterior limb of IC, while the inferior bundles of ML are returning via EC. The body of CC is labeled. VA enters the skull through the foramen magnum and is seen in the pontine cistern prior to joining the opposite VA to form the basilar artery.

CC	Corpus Callosum
CN	Caudate Nucleus
EC	External Capsule
GP	Globus Pallidus
IC	Internal Capsule
ICV	Internal Cerebral Vein
LV	Lateral Ventricle
MCP	Middle Cerebellar Peduncle
ML	Meyer's Loop
MO	Medulla Oblongata
OR	Optic Radiation
Pu	Putamen
RN	Red Nucleus
T	Thalamus
V3	Third Ventricle
VA	Vertebral Artery

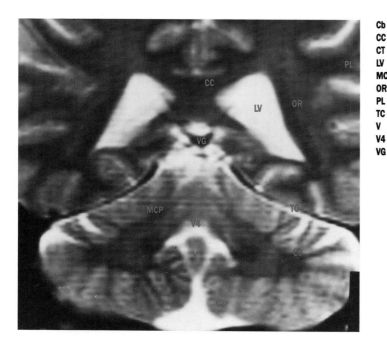

Cb	Cerebellum
CC	Corpus Callosum
CT	Cerebellar Tonsil
LV	Lateral Ventricle
MCP	Middle Cerebellar Peduncle
OR	Optic Radiation
PL	Parietal Lobe
TC	Tentorium Cerebelli
V	Vermis of Cerebellum
V4	Fourth Ventricle
VG	Vein of Galen

Figure 4-31 *T2-weighted, Optic Radiations at Level of Splenium of Corpus Callosum* This section is 16 mm posterior to Figure 4-30. LV is displaced laterally by the splenium of CC. Occlusion of the branches of the posterior cerebral artery, supplying the dominant occipital lobe and the splenium of the corpus callosum, can cause the syndrome of alexia without agraphia, in which written material perceived in the nondominant hemisphere cannot be transmitted via CC to the intact angular gyrus of PL. Because the angular gyrus is unaffected, these patients do not develop agraphia. OR is seen coursing laterally around LV within the retrolenticular portion of the internal capsule. TC is prominent on this T2-weighted image because it is outlined by cerebrospinal fluid. TC is a crescentic, arched, duplicated dural membrane that covers Cb and supports the occipital lobes. V extends through the posterior portion of the tentorial notch or incisura. TC is attached anteriorly at the posterior clinoid process. TC arises from a line of attachment along the inner margins of the occipital bone at the groove for the transverse sinus. VG (great cerebral vein) is formed by the merger of the internal cerebral veins (see Figure 4-10) and the basal veins of Rosenthal.

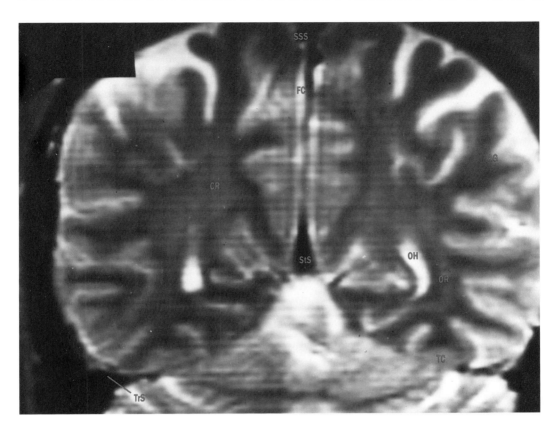

Figure 4-32 *T2-weighted, Occipital Horn of Lateral Ventricle* OH is seen within the parietal lobe. Lesions of the parietal lobe internal sagittal stratum (the white matter immediately adjacent to the lateral ventricle) are associated with defective optokinetic nystagmus. Lesions involving AG of the dominant hemisphere are associated with visual receptive aphasia, interfering with written language reception and production and causing both alexia and agraphia. CR is a fan-shaped structure comprised of myelinated projections of the internal capsule and other intrahemispheric tracts. FC is a sickle-shaped, duplicated dural membrane extending from the crista galli anteriorly to the internal occipital protuberance. FC lies in the interhemispheric fissure: SSS is located at the upper margin of FC, while StS is located in its lower margin at the junction with TC. TrS is located laterally in TC and drains venous blood anteriorly from the torcula to the sigmoid sinuses, eventually emptying into the internal jugular vein.

AG	Angular Gyrus of Parietal Lobe
CR	Corona Radiata
FC	Falx Cerebri
OH	Occipital Horn of Lateral Ventricle
OR	Optic Radiation
SSS	Superior Sagittal Sinus
StS	Straight Sinus
TC	Tentorium Cerebelli
TrS	Transverse Sinus

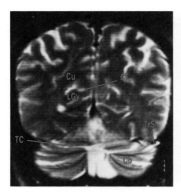 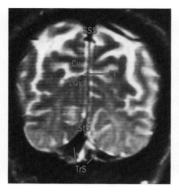 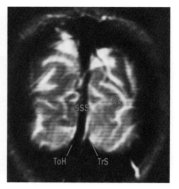

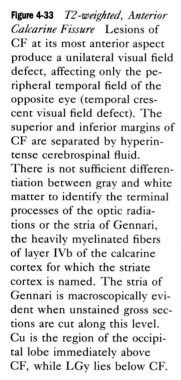

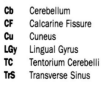

Figure 4-33 *T2-weighted, Anterior Calcarine Fissure* Lesions of CF at its most anterior aspect produce a unilateral visual field defect, affecting only the peripheral temporal field of the opposite eye (temporal crescent visual field defect). The superior and inferior margins of CF are separated by hyperintense cerebrospinal fluid. There is not sufficient differentiation between gray and white matter to identify the terminal processes of the optic radiations or the stria of Gennari, the heavily myelinated fibers of layer IVb of the calcarine cortex for which the striate cortex is named. The stria of Gennari is macroscopically evident when unstained gross sections are cut along this level. Cu is the region of the occipital lobe immediately above CF, while LGy lies below CF.

Cb	Cerebellum
CF	Calcarine Fissure
Cu	Cuneus
LGy	Lingual Gyrus
TC	Tentorium Cerebelli
TrS	Transverse Sinus

Figure 4-34 *T2-weighted, Posterior Calcarine Fissure* Except for the anterior aspect of CF, the primary visual cortex is binocularly innervated and most of its area is concerned with macular vision. The adjacent areas are the secondary or visual association areas. StS is seen emptying directly into the origin of the right TrS. As in this case, StS does not always contribute to the confluence of the sinuses (torcula), described in more detail with Figure 4-35.

CF	Calcarine Fissure
Cu	Cuneus
LGy	Lingual Gyrus
SSS	Superior Sagittal Sinus
StS	Straight Sinus
TrS	Transverse Sinus

Figure 4-35 *T2-weighted, Torcula* The primary visual cortex extends onto the posterior surface of OL and is not confined to the lips of the calcarine fissure, which is anterior to the plane of this section. The occipital pole is located in an arterial "watershed zone" between the regions supplied by the middle and posterior cerebral arteries. ToH is located at the internal occipital protuberance and is the confluence of SSS with the two transverse sinuses (TrS). Thrombosis of venous outflow from the brain can be detected by the absence of the normally seen venous flow void. This may be associated with pseudotumor cerebri.

OL	Occipital Lobe
SSS	Superior Sagittal Sinus
ToH	Torcula Heterophilus
TrS	Transverse Sinus

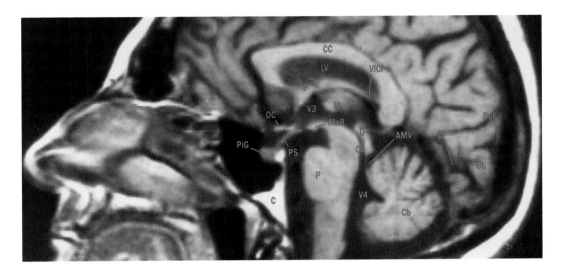

Figure 4-36 *T1-weighted, Midline* This section was imaged from a geriatric patient in whom cerebral atrophy allows better discrimination of the gyri and sulci than in younger patients (compare the oblique sagittal Figures 2-19 through 2-25). CF joins PoF posterior to the splenium of CC. The cuneus of OL lies between these two fissures. AMV is located in the roof of V4 and contains the decussating fibers of the trochlear nerve (see Figure 4-37). The posterior lobe of PiG is hyperintense because of fat present around the gland within the sella. Tumors of PiG must extend at least 10 mm superior to the sella before impinging on OC. The sella may be mostly filled with cerebrospinal fluid—an "empty sella." This can occur without any pathologic process or can result from increased intracranial pressure. Rarely, the optic nerves and chiasm may be displaced inferiorly into the sella. The syndrome of pituitary apoplexy results from sudden increase of intrasellar volume following hemorrhage into a tumor. MRI is particularly useful in these patients, whose symptoms can include severe pain and visual loss. The supraoptic recess of V3 is located above OC; it is bounded laterally on either side by the hypothalamus and anteriorly by the lamina terminalis. CA separates the tegmentum from the tectum of the midbrain, which contains Q, made up of the paired superior and inferior colliculi.

AMV	Anterior Medullary Velum
C	Clivus
CA	Cerebral Aqueduct
Cb	Cerebellum
CC	Corpus Callosum
CF	Calcarine Fissure
F	Fornix
IA	Interthalamic Adhesion
LV	Lateral Ventricle
MaB	Mamillary Body
OC	Optic Chiasm
OL	Occipital Lobe
P	Pons
PiG	Pituitary Gland
PoF	Parieto-occipital Fissure
PS	Pituitary Stalk
Q	Quadrigeminal Plate
V3	Third Ventricle
V4	Fourth Ventricle
VICi	Cistern of Velum Interpositum

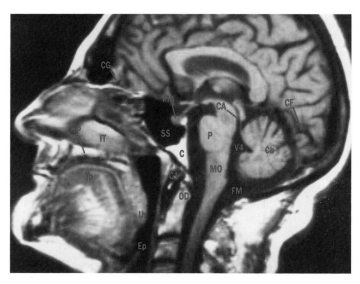

C	Clivus
C1	Atlas (1st Cervical Vertebra)
CA	Cerebral Aqueduct
Cb	Cerebellum
CF	Calcarine Fissure
CG	Crista Galli of Ethmoid Bone
Ep	Epiglottis
FM	Foramen Magnum
HP	Hard Palate
IT	Inferior Turbinate
MO	Medulla Oblongata
OD	Odontoid Process of C2
P	Pons
PiG	Pituitary Gland
SS	Sphenoid Sinus
To	Tongue
Uv	Uvula
V4	Fourth Ventricle

Figure 4-37 *T1-weighted, Midline* This image is identical to Figure 4-36. It is sized and cropped differently to allow labeling of the structures seen more inferiorly in the midsagittal plane. CG is the anterior inferior attachment of the falx cerebri. C1 may be congenitally fused with the base of the skull (atlanto-occipital fusion) and may be associated with deformities of FM, including basilar impression, a developmental deformity in which the cervical spine appears to push the occipital bone upward, and platybasia, a condition in which the basal angle of the skull is increased. Periodic alternating nystagmus, downbeat nystagmus, and other vertical eye movement disorders are associated with congenital and acquired abnormalities in the region of FM. These include the Arnold-Chiari malformation, in which the tonsils of Cb are displaced downward through FM. The midline sagittal MRI is now the standard method for diagnosing the Arnold-Chiari malformation. Basilar invagination, a condition in which the margins of FM are invaginated upward into the skull, is the result of softening of the bones of the skull base in conditions such as Paget's disease, osteogenesis imperfecta, osteomalacia, and hypoparathyroidism. Enlargement of MO and of the cervical spinal cord occurs in syringobulbia and syringomyelia. MRI is of great value in distinguishing intrinsic from extrinsic disorders of the brain stem in the region of FM.

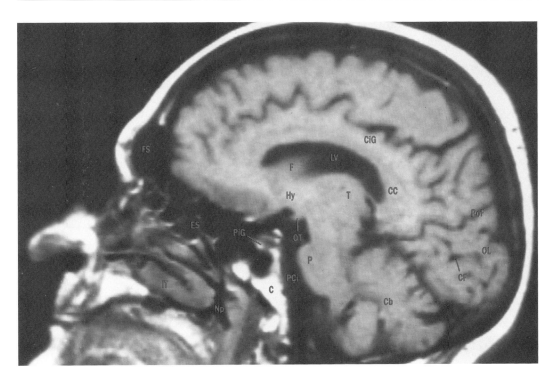

Figure 4-38 *T1-weighted, Parasagittal, 0.8 cm Lateral to Midline* CiG lies above CC and is separated from the remainder of the medial surfaces of the parietal and frontal lobes by the cingulate sulcus. PCi separates C from P.

C	Clivus
Cb	Cerebellum
CC	Corpus Callosum
CF	Calcarine Fissure
CiG	Cingulate Gyrus
ES	Ethmoid Sinus
F	Fornix
FS	Frontal Sinus
Hy	Hypothalamus
IT	Inferior Turbinate
LV	Lateral Ventricle
Np	Nasopharynx
OL	Occipital Lobe
OT	Optic Tract
P	Pons
PCi	Pontine Cistern
PiG	Pituitary Gland
PoF	Parieto-occipital Fissure
T	Thalamus

VESSELS AND CISTERNS

4-2-1 MRI: Angiography

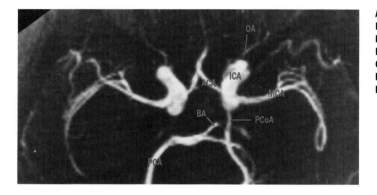

ACA	Anterior Cerebral Artery
BA	Basilar Artery
ICA	Internal Carotid Artery
MCA	Middle Cerebral Artery
OA	Ophthalmic Artery
PCA	Posterior Cerebral Artery
PCoA	Posterior Communicating Artery

Figure 4-39 *Axial* Compare this image to Figure 4-42. Note the superior resolution seen here compared to the CT image. This image can be rotated 360° to facilitate identifying structures and to eliminate overlap of structures. Figures 4-40 and 4-41 demonstrate different manipulations of this image.

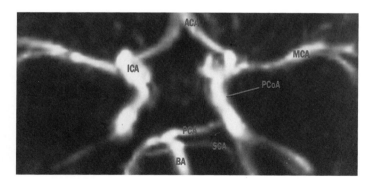

ACA	Anterior Cerebral Artery
BA	Basilar Artery
ICA	Internal Carotid Artery
MCA	Middle Cerebral Artery
PCA	Posterior Cerebral Artery
PCoA	Posterior Communicating Artery
SCA	Superior Cerebellar Artery

Figure 4-40 *Oblique Projection* This projection is sometimes called a *somersault* because it is rotated forward like a gymnast on a mat. It is obtained by taking an axial image as in Figure 4-39 and changing the angulation either positively or negatively, placing it more in the coronal plane. In this image, SCA can be discriminated from PCA because of the rotation.

SCA cannot be seen in the axial projection of Figure 4-39. The ophthalmic arteries cannot usually be seen on MRI angiography. The most common location of aneurysm causing oculomotor-nerve palsies is at the junction of PCoA and ICA. This location is seen well on this view.

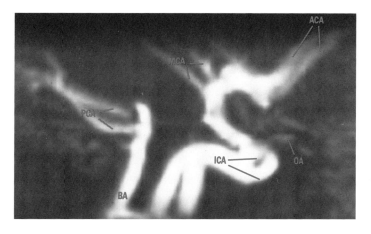

ACA	Anterior Cerebral Artery
BA	Basilar Artery
ICA	Internal Carotid Artery
MCA	Middle Cerebral Artery
OA	Ophthalmic Artery
PCA	Posterior Cerebral Artery

Figure 4-41 *Lateral Projection*
This projection is obtained by spinning the image around its central axis, producing a projection similar to a lateral conventional angiogram. This image is not quite rotated to the lateral projection, allowing separation of the vessels from their counterparts on the opposite side. A third MRI angiographic projection, not demonstrated here, is a horizontal projection. This is obtained by rotating the image on its side.

4-2-2 CT: Axial, Contrast-Enhanced

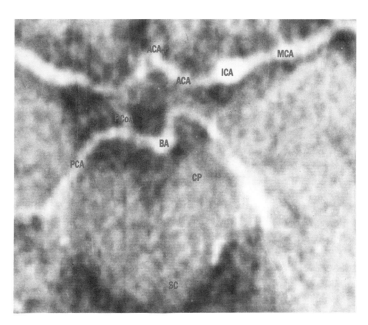

ACA	Anterior Cerebral Artery
ACA-P	Anterior Cerebral Artery— Pericallosal Branch
BA	Basilar Artery
CP	Cerebral Peduncle
ICA	Internal Carotid Artery
MCA	Middle Cerebral Artery
PCA	Posterior Cerebral Artery
PCoA	Posterior Communicating Artery
SC	Superior Colliculus

Figure 4-42 *Arterial Circle of Willis* Compare this image to the axial MRI angiogram (Figure 4-39). The resolution of CT does not enable visualization of small aneurysms. The appearance of an aneurysm on MRI relates to whether clotting and leakage of blood have occurred.

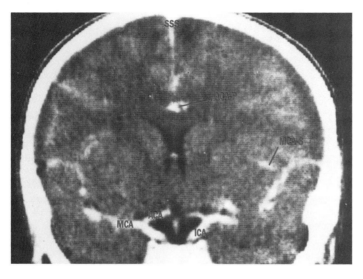

ACA	Anterior Cerebral Artery
ACA-P	Anterior Cerebral Artery— Pericallosal Branch
ICA	Internal Carotid Artery
MCA	Middle Cerebral Artery
MCA-S	Middle Cerebral Artery—Sylvian Branch
SSS	Superior Sagittal Sinus

Figure 4-43 *Anterior and Middle Cerebral Arteries* Coronal views may be helpful in following the branching pattern of ACA and MCA. The suprasellar portion of ICA bifurcates into ACA and MCA.

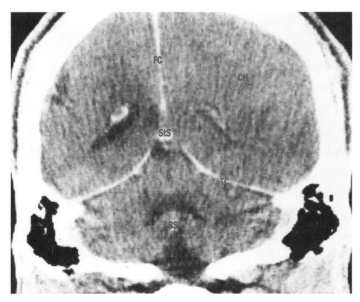

BS	Brain Stem
CH	Cerebral Hemisphere
FC	Falx Cerebri
StS	Straight Sinus
TC	Tentorium Cerebelli
V	Vermis of Cerebellum
V4	Fourth Ventricle

Figure 4-44 *Straight Sinus* The posterior fossa lies below TC. TC is attached to FC at the midline and descends to its lateral attachment at the superior margin of the petrous part of the temporal bone. The superior part of V may lie superior to the inferior surface of CH. StS is at the junction of TC and FC.

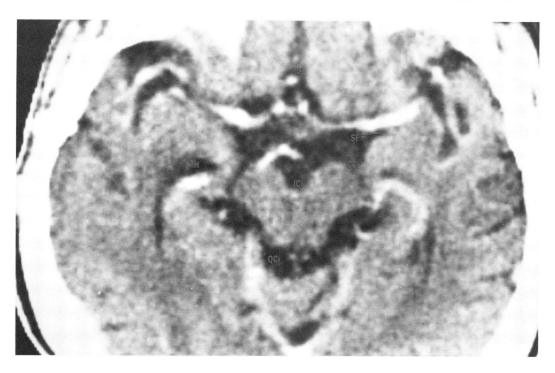

Figure 4-45 *Suprasellar Cistern and Its Extensions* This image demonstrates the cisterns well because of cerebral atrophy, which allows for dilation of the cisterns. The intracranial optic nerves, optic chiasm, and optic tracts are located in the suprasellar cistern. This cistern is pentagonal in its axial plane, or (if one adds ICi into considera- tion) it may be viewed as hav- ing 6 extensions or "points," making the star-shaped outline seen here. IF is the most ante- rior point. The anterolateral points are the medial aspects of SF and separate the uncus of the temporal lobe from the inferomedial part of the frontal lobe. The posterolateral points extend into CCi. ICi makes up the sixth and most posterior point.

CCi	Crural Cistern
ICi	Interpeduncular Cistern
IF	Interhemispheric Fissure
QCi	Quadrigeminal Plate Cistern
SF	Sylvian Fissure
TH	Temporal Horn of Lateral Ventricle

CHAPTER 5

Afferent Visual Pathway

OPTIC NERVE, INTRAORBITAL

5-1-1 MRI: Axial

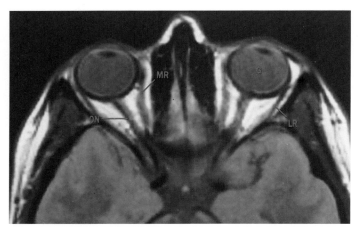

G Globe
LR Lateral Rectus Muscle
MR Medial Rectus Muscle
ON Optic Nerve

Figure 5-1 *Proton-Density-weighted, Chemical Shift Artifact* This is a proton-density-weighted (first-echo) image. Note the black line surrounding G and coursing back along ON. This is an example of chemical shift artifact, a signal created by the different resonant frequencies of fat and water. The signal of the fat molecules is artificially darkened on one side, where relatively water-rich soft tissue interfaces with fat. Elimination of this artifact requires using a smaller acquisition pixel size (sampling smaller areas yields greater accuracy) or using fat-suppression techniques (see Figure 5-2).

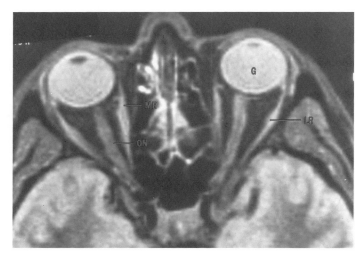

G Globe
LR Lateral Rectus Muscle
MR Medial Rectus Muscle
ON Optic Nerve

Figure 5-2 *Fat-Suppressed Correction of Chemical Shift Artifact* This is a STIR image of the same orbit seen in Figure 5-1. Note the homogeneity of the fat on either side of ON and G. There is still a hypointense area surrounding the fat–water interface, but it is symmetric.

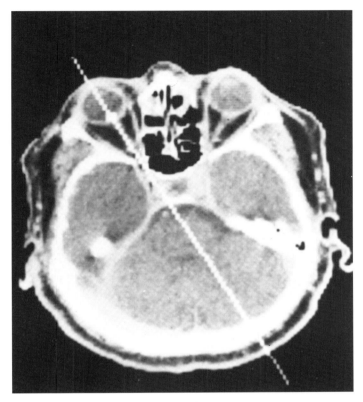

IR   Inferior Rectus Muscle
ON   Optic Nerve
SR   Superior Rectus Muscle

Figure 5-3 *Intraorbital Optic Nerve* Off-axis computer re-formatting in this plane provides a lateral view of the orbital contents. This enables delineation of SR and IR from the orbital walls. The line in the axial image indicates the plane of the reformatted image. This technique is rarely used today; it has been superseded by direct sagittal MRI. Direct sagittal CT imaging of the orbit is possible, but requires awkward positioning of the patient within the scanner.

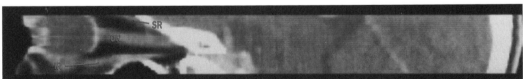

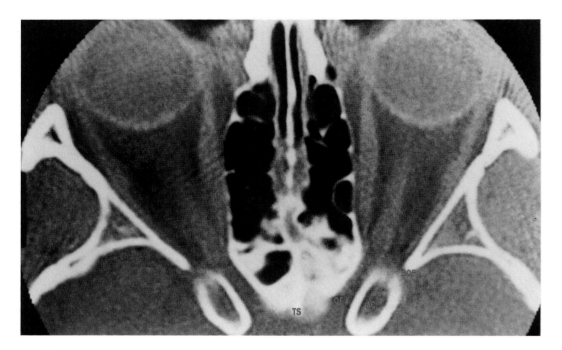

Figure 5-4 *Optic Foramen* To achieve this image, thin, properly angulated sections must be used or the section will include part of the bony roof or floor of OF. OF is medial to AC, while SOF is anterolateral to AC. Note that the posterior portion of OF is wider than the anterior portion on this slice. Anteriorly, OF has a long vertical axis, while posteriorly its long axis is horizontal. Anatomically, this corresponds to the location of the ophthalmic artery, which is lateral to the optic nerve posteriorly and superior to it anteriorly. The intracanalicular portion of the optic nerve is seen in sagittal section in MRI Figure 2-23. TS is often the origin of meningiomas invading OF or compressing the optic nerve or optic chiasm from below.

AC	Anterior Clinoid
OF	Optic Foramen
SOF	Superior Orbital Fissure
TS	Tuberculum Sellae

OPTIC NERVE, INTRACRANIAL

5-2-1 CT: Axial, Contrast-Enhanced

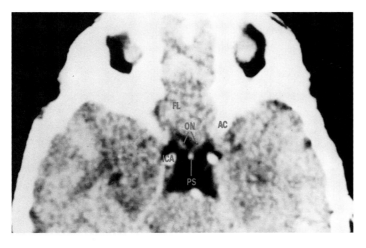

AC	Anterior Clinoid
FL	Frontal Lobe
ICA	Internal Carotid Artery
ON	Optic Nerve
PS	Pituitary Stalk

optic foramen is not seen because ON also shifts superiorly (at a 45° angle from the horizontal plane) on its way to the chiasm; thus, the optic foramen is inferior to the plane of this image.

Figure 5-5 *Intracranial Optic Nerve* ON passes posteriorly and medially from the optic foramen (compare the more lateral position of the intracanalicular ON in Figure 5-4). The

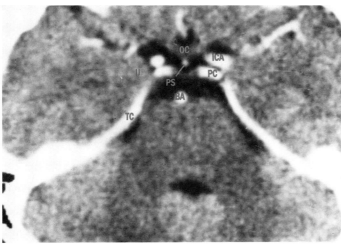

BA	Basilar Artery
ICA	Internal Carotid Artery
OC	Optic Chiasm
PC	Posterior Clinoid
PS	Pituitary Stalk
TC	Tentorium Cerebelli
U	Uncus of Temporal Lobe

Figure 5-6 *Optic Nerve Joining Optic Chiasm* In this figure, superior to Figure 5-5, the optic nerves are seen joining OC. This image would be helpful in assessing a junctional visual field defect, where the lesion involves the intracranial optic nerve and OC.

OPTIC CHIASM

5-3-1 MRI: Axial

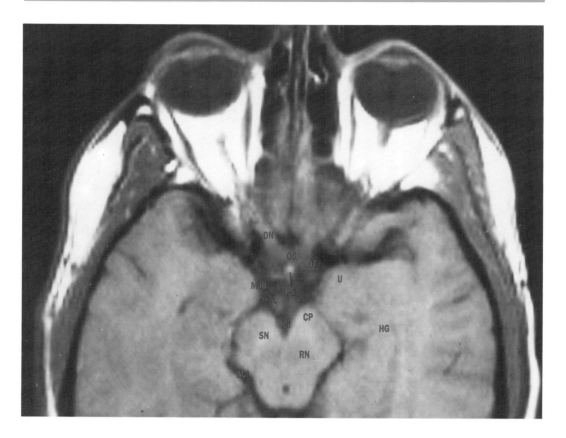

Figure 5-7 *T1-weighted, Optic Chiasm* This section is at a level between the superior and inferior colliculi in the tectum of the midbrain. The intra-axial (intra–brain-stem) fibers of the oculomotor nerve course from their origin in the oculo-

motor nucleus through the mesencephalic tegmentum through RN and CP. ACi is seen in its circummesence-phalic location anterior to and continuous with the quadri-geminal plate cistern. MaB is a prominent structure be-tween PS and the midbrain.

ACi	Ambient Cistern
CP	Cerebral Peduncle
HG	Hippocampal Gyrus
ICi	Interpeduncular Cistern
MaB	Mamillary Body
OC	Optic Chiasm
ON	Optic Nerve
OT	Optic Tract
PS	Pituitary Stalk
RN	Red Nucleus
SN	Substantia Nigra
U	Uncus of Temporal Lobe

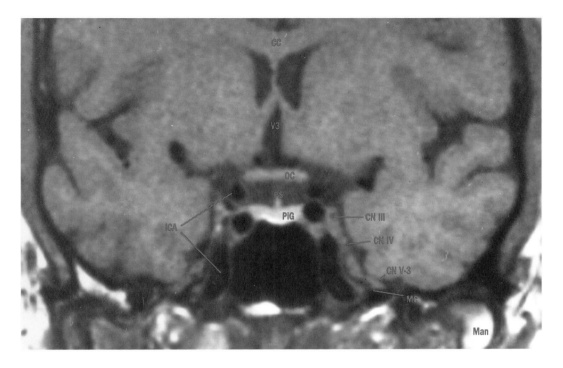

Figure 5-8 *T1-weighted, Optic Chiasm* This figure and text are identical to Figure 4-20 and are repeated here for continuity. The intracavernous ICA is seen both in longitudinal and in cross sections because of its S-shaped course (compare with the sagittal view, Figure 2-24). ICA is also seen in the suprasellar cistern, inferolateral to OC. CN V-3 is seen as it exits MC and passes into the foramen ovale (compare with the CT in Figure 2-47). The supraoptic recess of V3 is seen above OC. Bitemporal hemianopia is the hallmark of chiasmal dysfunction. If compression of OC comes from below, the field defect begins superiorly and progresses in a clockwise direction in the right visual field and in a counterclockwise direction in the left. PiG lies approximately 10 mm below the chiasm. Before visual field defects become apparent, pituitary adenomas must be large enough to break through the diaphragma sellae and extend into the suprasellar cistern, where they compress the visual pathway. If OC is compressed from above, as in a craniopharyngioma, the inferior temporal fields may be the first affected.

CC	Corpus Callosum
CN III	Oculomotor Nerve
CN IV	Trochlear Nerve
CN V-3	Trigeminal Nerve—3rd Division
ICA	Internal Carotid Artery
Man	Mandible
MC	Meckel's Cave
OC	Optic Chiasm
PiG	Pituitary Gland
PS	Pituitary Stalk
V3	Third Ventricle

5-3 Optic Chiasm **143**

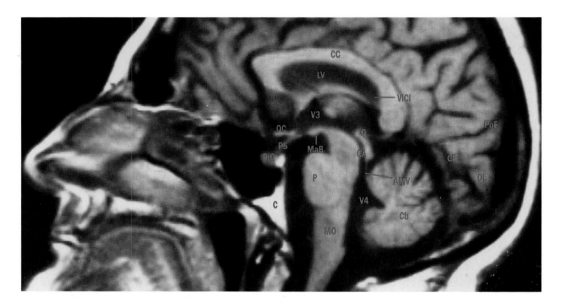

Figure 5-9 *T1-weighted, Optic Chiasm* This figure is derived from Figure 4-36 and is included here for continuity. This section was imaged from a geriatric patient in whom cerebral atrophy allows better discrimination of the gyri and sulci than in younger patients (compare the oblique sagittal Figures 2-19 through 2-25). CF joins PoF posterior to the splenium of CC. The cuneus of OL lies between these two fissures. AMV is located in the roof of V4 and contains the decussating fibers of the trochlear nerve. The posterior lobe of PiG is hyperintense because of fat present around the gland within the sella. Tumors of PiG must extend at least 10 mm superior to the sella before

impinging on OC. OC is directly over the sella turcica in this figure, as it is in 80% of the population. It may be over the tuberculum sellae (prefixed) in 9% or over the dorsum sellae (postfixed) in 11%. This affects the angulation of the intracranial optic nerve and the resultant visual field defects. A postfixed OC may be involved with less extension of a tumor that arose in the sella. The supraoptic recess of V3 is located above OC; it is bounded laterally on either side by the hypothalamus and anteriorly by the lamina terminalis. CA separates the tegmentum from the tectum of the midbrain, which contains Q, made up of the paired superior and inferior colliculi.

AMV	Anterior Medullary Velum
C	Clivus
CA	Cerebral Aqueduct
Cb	Cerebellum
CC	Corpus Callosum
CF	Calcarine Fissure
LV	Lateral Ventricle
MaB	Mamillary Body
MO	Medulla Oblongata
OC	Optic Chiasm
OL	Occipital Lobe
P	Pons
PiG	Pituitary Gland
PoF	Parieto-occipital Fissure
PS	Pituitary Stalk
Q	Quadrigeminal Plate
V3	Third Ventricle
V4	Fourth Ventricle
VICI	Cistern of Velum Interpositum

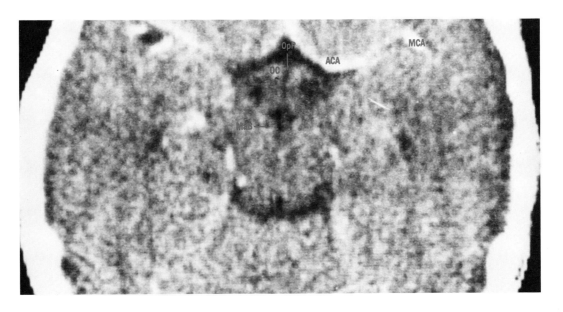

Figure 5-10 *Optic Chiasm* OC has a slit-like lucency in the middle due to low-density cerebrospinal fluid in OpR. OT is seen extending posteriorly from OC. MaB is seen within the hypothalamus, posterior to OC. OC is isodense with brain. Note ACA and MCA have branched off the internal carotid artery after it has exited the cavernous sinus (see Figure 5-5 for the location of the internal carotid artery).

ACA	Anterior Cerebral Artery
MaB	Mamillary Body
MCA	Middle Cerebral Artery
OC	Optic Chiasm
OpR	Optic Recess of Third Ventricle
OT	Optic Tract

OPTIC TRACT

5-4-1 MRI: Coronal

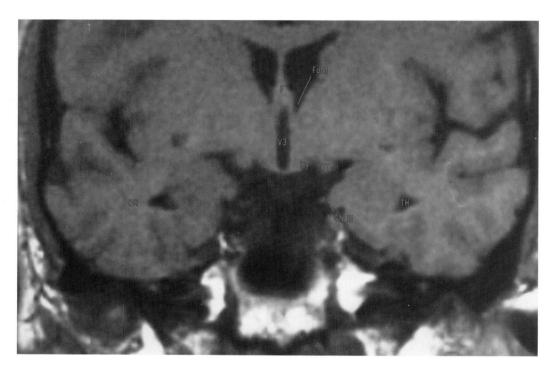

Figure 5-11 *T1-weighted, Optic Tract* This figure and text are identical to Figure 4-23 and are repeated here for continuity. OT is more lateral than in Figure 5-10 as it approaches the lateral geniculate body. Note the relationship of U to CN III. Herniation of the temporal lobe at this location may give rise to a dilated pupil (Hutchinson's pupil). This is the most anterior image containing TH. Following their exit from the lateral geniculate body, the in-ferior bundles of OR pass through the external sagittal stratum laterally and anteriorly and loop (Meyer's loop) around the tip of TH, where they turn posteriorly. The most anterior extent occurs at a point less than 1 cm lateral to the tip of TH. This is about 5 cm posterior to the tip of the temporal lobe. Anterior lesions of OT may result in noncongruous hemianopias because corresponding fibers from the two optic nerves do not occupy identical positions within OT at this location.

CN III	Oculomotor Nerve
F	Fornix
FoM	Foramen of Monro
Hy	Hypothalamus
OR	Optic Radiation
OT	Optic Tract
TH	Temporal Horn of Lateral Ventricle
U	Uncus of Temporal Lobe
V3	Third Ventricle

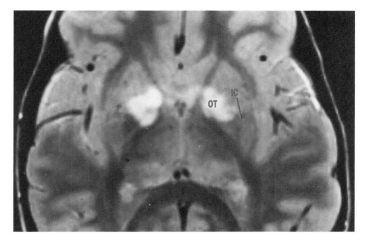

IC   Internal Capsule
OT   Optic Tract

Figure 5-12 *Proton-Density-weighted, Optic Tract* This OT is naturally enhanced in a patient with a hamartoma of the anterior visual pathway, which is frequently associated with an anterior visual pathway (optic nerve and optic chiasm) glioma. In this image, the posterior termination of OT at the lateral geniculate body is hyperintense. Normally, OT cannot be differentiated from the adjacent white matter. The exception occurs when the ratio of water to fat is increased in OT. When anterior visual pathway gliomas extend backward from the optic chiasm into the diencephalon, they may take on the appearance of a pair of ice tongs surrounding the cerebral peduncles. The hamartoma serves to mark the course of OT, making it look falsely large. This is a proton-density-weighted (or first-echo T2-weighted) image. When tumors are surrounded by edema fluid, MRI shows hyperintensity on proton-density-weighted and T2-weighted images. Often, the edema cannot be differentiated from the substance of the tumor.

5-4-3 CT: Axial, Contrast-Enhanced

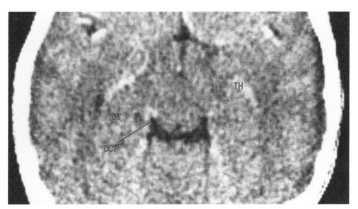

CCi   Crural Cistern
OT   Optic Tract
TH   Temporal Horn of Lateral Ventricle

Figure 5-13 *Optic Tract* OT is not identifiable, but its location is depicted lateral to CCi. Note the enhancement of the choroid plexus of TH with contrast.

LATERAL GENICULATE BODY

5-5-1 MRI: Coronal

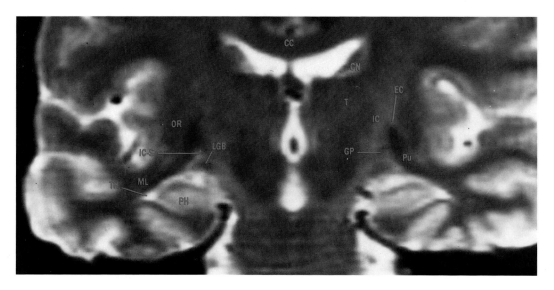

Figure 5-14 *T2-weighted, Lateral Geniculate Body* This slice is identical to Figure 4-29. LGB is difficult to image because it is a small structure composed of both gray and white matter, both of which are present in adjacent structures that are more easily identified. PH of the temporal lobe is below LGB and separated from it by the choroidal fissure. GP and Pu (together known as the *lentiform nucleus*) are above LGB, from which they are separated by IC-S. The posterior limb of IC forms the medial border of the lentiform nucleus, while the lateral border is formed by EC. The axons that comprise OR arise from LGB and enter IC-S and the posterior (or retrolenticular) limb of IC. The upper (dorsal) fibers of OR (at the location labeled) originate in the medial aspect of LGB and pass almost vertically into IC, while the ventral fibers of OR pass laterally and inferiorly through the temporal lobe as ML, where they loop posteriorly, finally returning to IC. LGB derives its arterial supply from the anterior and posterior choroidal arteries. Insufficiency of blood supply from the anterior choroidal artery may cause congruous superior and inferior homonymous hemianopias, whereas insufficiency of blood supply from the posterior choroidal artery may cause horizontal homonymous sectoranopias.

CC	Corpus Callosum
CN	Caudate Nucleus
EC	External Capsule
GP	Globus Pallidus
IC	Internal Capsule
IC-S	Internal Capsule—Sublentiform Portion
LGB	Lateral Geniculate Body
ML	Meyer's Loop
OR	Optic Radiation
PH	Pes Hippocampus
Pu	Putamen
T	Thalamus
TH	Temporal Horn of Lateral Ventricle

OPTIC RADIATIONS

5-6-1 CT: Axial, Contrast-Enhanced

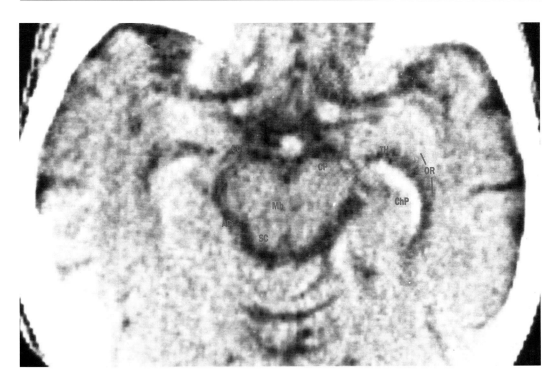

Figure 5-15 *Optic Radiation, Inferior Temporal Lobe* OR (the geniculocalcarine tract) is located in white matter of the internal capsule just lateral to TH. The fibers of the internal capsule are described in relation to the lateral ventricle. The closest fibers comprise the internal sagittal stratum, and the more peripheral fibers are the external sagittal stratum, which contains OR. ChP is seen enhanced within TH. CCi outlines CP (crus cerebri) and continues posteriorly as ACi, which then courses along the tentorium cerebelli. The name *crural cistern* originates from its location lateral to the crus cerebri (CP).

ACi	Ambient Cistern
CCi	Crural Cistern
ChP	Choroid Plexus
CP	Cerebral Peduncle
Mb	Midbrain
OR	Optic Radiation
SC	Superior Colliculus
TH	Temporal Horn of Lateral Ventricle

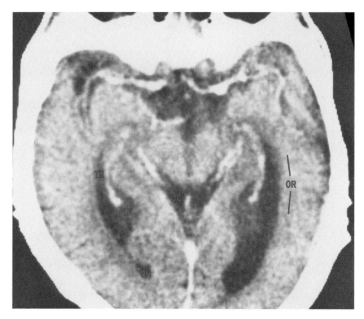

LV	Lateral Ventricle—Trigone
OH	Occipital Horn of Lateral Ventricle
OR	Optic Radiation
QCi	Quadrigeminal Plate Cistern
TH	Temporal Horn of Lateral Ventricle

Figure 5-16 *Optic Radiation, Negative Angulation* This slice is at the level of the tentorial incisura. The ventricles and cisterns are seen well because of cerebral atrophy. The inferior portion of OR passes superior and lateral to TH and extends to the inferior tip of the calcarine fissure within the inferior longitudinal fasciculus. *Quadrigeminal plate* refers to the dorsal or tectal part of the midbrain, containing the superior and inferior colliculi.

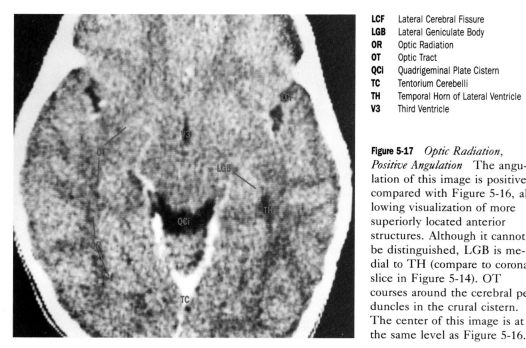

LCF	Lateral Cerebral Fissure
LGB	Lateral Geniculate Body
OR	Optic Radiation
OT	Optic Tract
QCi	Quadrigeminal Plate Cistern
TC	Tentorium Cerebelli
TH	Temporal Horn of Lateral Ventricle
V3	Third Ventricle

Figure 5-17 *Optic Radiation, Positive Angulation* The angulation of this image is positive compared with Figure 5-16, allowing visualization of more superiorly located anterior structures. Although it cannot be distinguished, LGB is medial to TH (compare to coronal slice in Figure 5-14). OT courses around the cerebral peduncles in the crural cistern. The center of this image is at the same level as Figure 5-16.

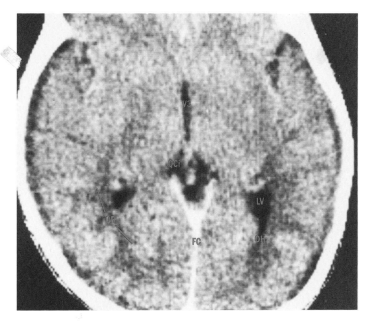

FC	Falx Cerebri
LV	Lateral Ventricle—Trigone
OH	Occipital Horn of Lateral Ventricle
OR	Optic Radiation
QCi	Quadrigeminal Plate Cistern
V3	Third Ventricle

Figure 5-18 *Optic Radiation, Calcarine Fissure* This section is at the approximate level of the calcarine fissure of the occipital lobe, although the fissure cannot be distinguished. QCi is seen anterior to FC, which separates the occipital lobes. This image shows more of V3 within the subthalamus than does Figure 5-17.

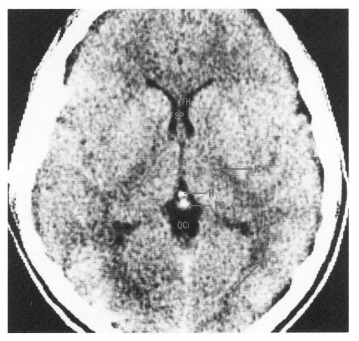

FH	Frontal Horn of Lateral Ventricle
H	Habenula
IC	Internal Capsule
OR	Optic Radiation
PG	Pineal Gland
QCi	Quadrigeminal Plate Cistern
SP	Septum Pellucidum
T	Thalamus
V3	Third Ventricle

Figure 5-19 *Optic Radiation and Pineal Gland* SP separates the two lateral ventricles. Absence of SP may be seen associated with optic nerve hypoplasia in deMorsier's syndrome. V3 separates the thalami; occasionally, there are intrathalamic adhesions, termed *massa intermedia*. H and PG are calcified and lie posteriorly in V3. The course of OR is indicated with lines.

CHAPTER 6

Sella and Parasellar Structures

SELLA TURCICA

6-1-1 CT: Axial, Contrast-Enhanced

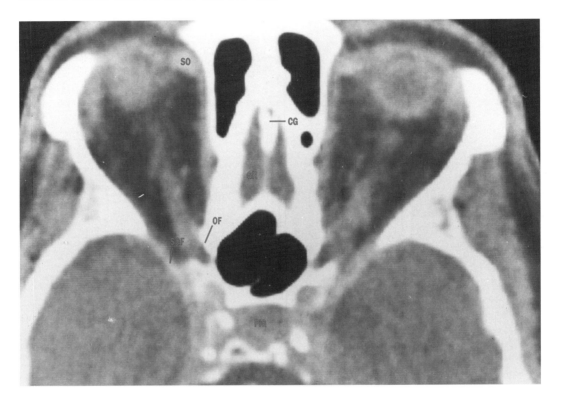

Figure 6-1 *Sellar Contents* At the apex of the orbit, SOF is seen lateral to OF. This slice is taken parallel to the orbito-meatal line; as a result, only the more superiorly located posterior part of OF is seen (Figure 2-28 shows a slice through the entire OF). Note the proximity of the optic nerves to PiG as the nerves enter the intracranial space, near the chiasm. The olfactory bulb and tract run within the olfactory sulcus lateral to GR (see Figures 2-13 and 2-14). The olfactory groove of the cribriform plate of the ethmoid bone is slightly inferior to the plane of this section and contains the olfactory bulb. Meningiomas involving the olfactory groove may cause the Foster Kennedy syndrome of ipsilateral optic atrophy, contralateral papilledema, and ipsilateral anosmia.

CG	Crista Galli of Ethmoid Bone
GR	Gyrus Rectus of Frontal Lobe
OF	Optic Foramen
PiG	Pituitary Gland
SO	Superior Oblique Muscle
SOF	Superior Orbital Fissure

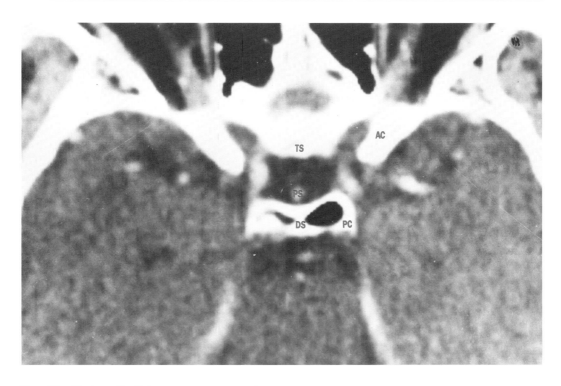

Figure 6-2 *Pituitary Stalk in Suprasellar Cistern* Because both AC and PC are seen, this section is at or above the level of the diaphragma sellae. Note the enhancement of PS. The free tips of AC extend medially, whereas the free tips of PC extend laterally. TS and DS are the landmarks that define a prefixed and a postfixed optic chiasm, respectively.

AC Anterior Clinoid
DS Dorsum Sellae
PC Posterior Clinoid
PS Pituitary Stalk
TS Tuberculum Sellae

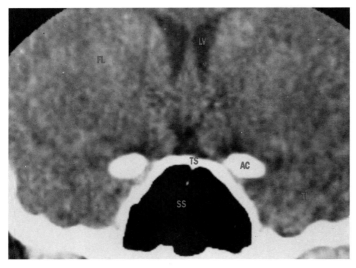

AC	Anterior Clinoid
FL	Frontal Lobe
LV	Lateral Ventricle
SS	Sphenoid Sinus
TL	Temporal Lobe
TS	Tuberculum Sellae

Figure 6-3 *Tuberculum Sellae* AC is lateral to TS. The optic nerves lie below but cannot be distinguished from the gyrus rectus of the adjacent FL and are not easily visualized until they enter the suprasellar (chiasmatic) cistern.

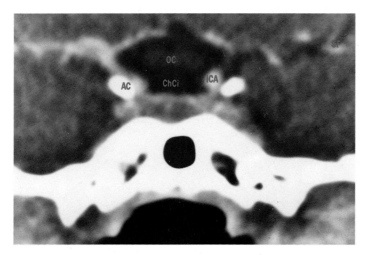

AC	Anterior Clinoid
ChCi	Chiasmatic Cistern
ICA	Internal Carotid Artery
OC	Optic Chiasm
SF	Sylvian Fissure

Figure 6-4 *Optic Chiasm* This figure is imaged with a window to best demonstrate OC. Within ChCi, the optic nerves join to form OC, where they create a dumbbell shape.

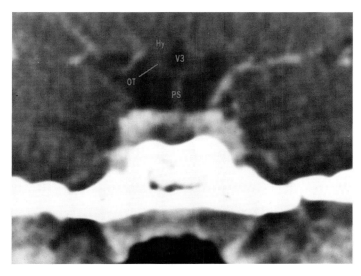

Hy	Hypothalamus
OT	Optic Tract
PS	Pituitary Stalk
V3	Third Ventricle

Figure 6-5 *Optic Tract* The infundibular recess is the inferior extension of V3 into Hy. OT extends back alongside Hy. PS extends inferiorly from Hy into the sella.

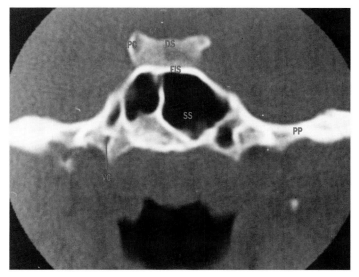

DS	Dorsum Sellae
FIS	Floor of Sella
PC	Posterior Clinoid
PP	Petrous Pyramid of Temporal Bone
SS	Sphenoid Sinus
VC	Vidian Canal

Figure 6-6 *Dorsum Sellae* The window setting of this image was chosen to optimize bony detail. The oculomotor nerve (not seen) grooves the lateral aspect of DS and courses above the superior aspect of the cavernous sinus before entering the cavernous sinus anterior to the plane of this section.

CAVERNOUS SINUS

6-2-1 MRI: Coronal

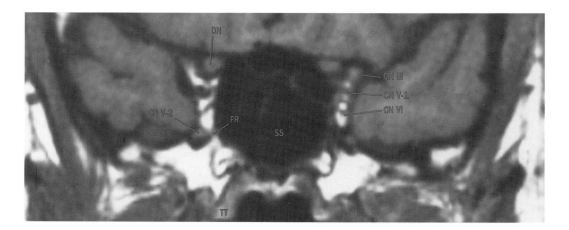

Figure 6-7 *T1-weighted, Cavernous Sinus* This figure is derived from Figure 4-18 and is included here for continuity. The intracavernous course of CN III, IV, V, and VI is distinguished more clearly on MRI than CT (compare Figure 6-8). CN IV is inferolateral to CN III, but cannot be delineated because of its small size, only 3400 axons. CN V-1 lies below CN III. CN V-1 divides into three branches in the most anterior part of the cavernous sinus, the largest of which is the frontal nerve. CN V-2 has already departed from the cavernous sinus and is seen as a separate structure below the cavernous sinus, in FR. The nerves cannot be labeled with certainty because of their shifting relationships within the cavernous sinus. Note the su-peromedial course of ON as it passes from the orbit into the brain. At this level, it is difficult to be certain whether all borders of ON are within the optic foramen, in which case ON is separated from the cavernous sinus contents by the optic strut of the sphenoid bone. Posterior to the point where the inferior border of ON exits the optic foramen, the superior border is covered by a layer of dura, the falciform fold. On T1-weighted scans, the sphenoid bone, air in SS, and dura forming the falciform fold overlying the nerve all have a similar appearance. TT (or tubal elevation) is comprised of cartilage arising from the medial pterygoid process; it marks the nasopharyngeal opening of the auditory (eustachian) tube.

CN III	Oculomotor Nerve
CN V-1	Trigeminal Nerve—1st Division
CN V-2	Trigeminal Nerve—2nd Division
CN VI	Abducens Nerve
FR	Foramen Rotundum
ON	Optic Nerve
SS	Sphenoid Sinus
TT	Torus Tubarius

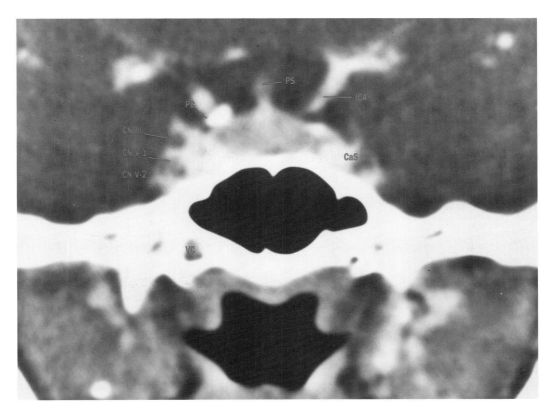

Figure 6-8 *Cavernous Sinus* This section is relatively posterior at the level of PS and catches the anterior tip of one PC (compare Figure 6-2). CaS is the enhanced structure seen lateral to the sella and sphenoid sinus. The cranial nerves appear as lucencies within CaS. CN III is the most superior and most consistently seen. The trochlear nerve is just below CN III, but may not be seen due to its small size. CN V-2 is seen only in caudal sections of CaS. ICA and the abducens nerve lie within CaS and are not seen separately. This anatomy is dramatically more distinct on coronal MRI (see Figure 6-7).

CaS	Cavernous Sinus
CN III	Oculomotor Nerve
CN V-1	Trigeminal Nerve—1st Division
CN V-2	Trigeminal Nerve—2nd Division
ICA	Internal Carotid Artery
PC	Posterior Clinoid
PS	Pituitary Stalk
VC	Vidian Canal

CHAPTER 7

Temporal Bone, Base of Skull, and Cranial Nerves

FACIAL NERVE

7-1-1 CT: Axial, Bone Window

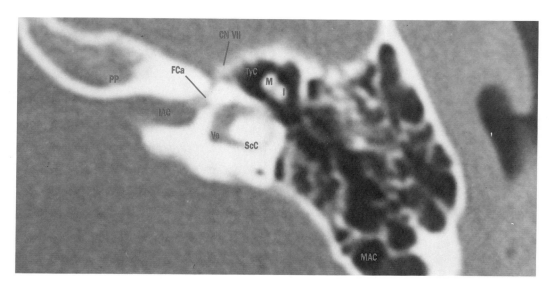

Figure 7-1 *Facial Nerve and Internal Auditory Canal* CN VII traverses the lateral pontine cistern prior to entering IAC (compare Figure 4-29). The motor root and nervus intermedius (sensory and parasympathetic fibers) of CN VII, along with the vestibulocochlear nerve and the internal auditory artery, enter the temporal bone through IAC. At the distal end of IAC, CN VII and VIII separate, with CN VII entering FCa. FCa is described as following a Z-shaped course of 28 to 30 mm divided into three segments. The first (labyrinthine) segment runs 4 mm from the termination of IAC to the geniculate ganglion. This ganglion is named for the sharp bend (first genu) in FCa at which it is located. The greater superficial petrosal nerve branches off CN VII just proximal to the geniculate ganglion. It then runs forward along PP toward the vidian canal, eventually innervating the lacrimal gland. The second (tympanic or horizontal) segment of FCa begins at the geniculate ganglion, along the medial wall of TyC. This segment runs for 11 mm, ending at the second genu of FCa. The third (mastoid or vertical) segment turns vertically and continues downward for 13 mm before exiting FCa through the stylomastoid foramen.

CN VII	Facial Nerve
FCa	Facial Canal
I	Incus
IAC	Internal Auditory Canal
M	Malleus
MAC	Mastoid Air Cells
PP	Petrous Pyramid of Temporal Bone
ScC	Semicircular Canal
TyC	Tympanic Cavity
Ve	Vestibule

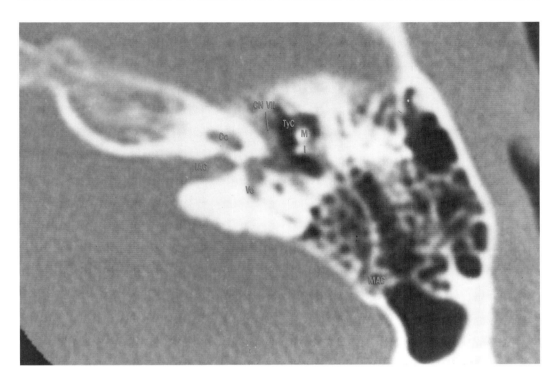

Figure 7-2 *Facial Nerve, 2nd Segment* This section is 3 mm inferior to Figure 7-1. After a sharp turn (first genu), the second (tympanic or horizontal) segment of CN VII begins at the geniculate ganglion and runs posteriorly in the medial wall of TyC (middle ear), from which it exits below the horizontal semicircular canals, where it turns at a right angle (second genu), becoming the third (mastoid or vertical) segment. The second segment of CN VII is seen in the coronal plane in Figure 7-3.

CN VII	Facial Nerve—2nd Segment
Co	Cochlea
I	Incus
IAC	Internal Auditory Canal
M	Malleus
MAC	Mastoid Air Cells
TyC	Tympanic Cavity
Ve	Vestibule

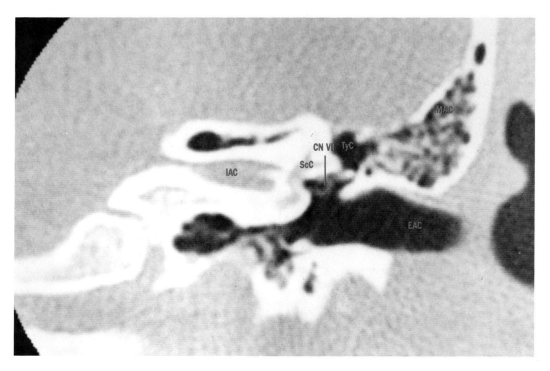

Figure 7-3 *Facial Nerve, 2nd Segment* The second segment of CN VII lies immediately below ScC. TyC is continuous with the pharynx via the auditory tube. Because of the air on both sides of TyC, pressure on either side of the tympanic membrane can be equilibrated.

CN VII	Facial Nerve—2nd Segment
EAC	External Auditory Canal
IAC	Internal Auditory Canal
MAC	Mastoid Air Cells
ScC	Semicircular Canal
TyC	Tympanic Cavity

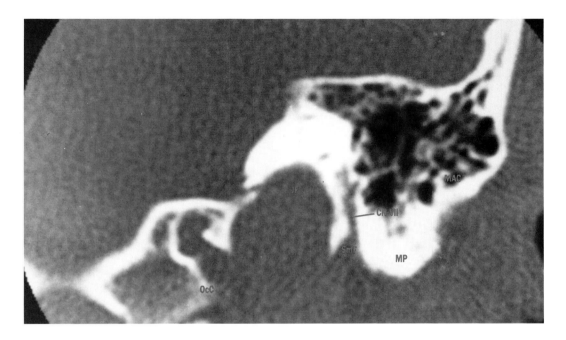

Figure 7-4 *Facial Nerve, 3rd Segment* This image is 5 mm posterior to Figure 7-3. After another sharp bend (second genu), the third (mastoid or vertical) segment of CN VII runs inferiorly to exit the skull base at SmF. Two branches are given off the facial nerve in the vertical portion of the facial canal: the first is the nerve to the stapedius muscle; the second is the chorda tympani. Paresis of the stapedial nerve may allow sounds to be perceived as too loud in the affected ear, and activity of fibers to this branch may cause patients to experience rustling sounds during facial contractions in hemifacial spasm. The chorda tympani is the second (and last) branch of the nervus intermedius, the first being the greater superficial petrosal nerve. The chorda tympani contains parasympathetic fibers for the submandibular gland and taste fibers for the anterior two thirds of the tongue. Surgery to decompress the facial canal is performed in some cases of Bell's palsy. Severe compression by edema can lead to aberrant regeneration of the facial nerve. This can cause gustatory lacrimation (crocodile tears) or synkinesis, with cocontracture of various facial muscles. Note that a needle directed toward CN VII at SmF for a Nadbath block could encounter the jugular vein and lead to hemorrhage at the skull base or anesthesia of the glossopharyngeal, vagus, and accessory nerves, which exit the skull within JF.

CN VII	Facial Nerve—3rd Segment
JF	Jugular Foramen
MAC	Mastoid Air Cells
MP	Mastoid Process of Temporal Bone
OcC	Occipital Condyle
SmF	Stylomastoid Foramen

BASE OF SKULL

7-2-1 CT: Axial, Bone Window

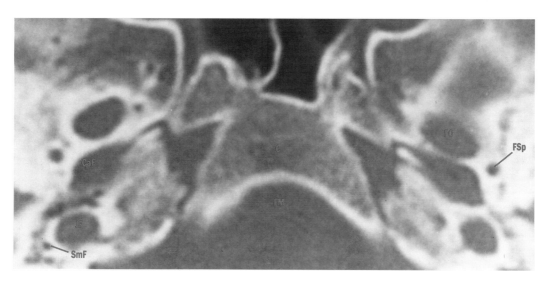

Figure 7-5 *Jugular and Other Basilar Foramina* SmF, the termination of the facial canal, is lateral to JF and transmits CN VII and the stylomastoid artery. JF lies posterior to CaF and transmits the glossopharyngeal, vagus, and accessory nerves, as well as the internal jugular vein and some meningeal artery branches. Knowledge of this anatomy is important if the facial nerve is to be blocked near the skull base with local anesthetic. For example, severe difficulty in breathing may result if the contralateral vocal cord had been previously paralyzed and the branches to the recurrent laryngeal nerve supplying the ipsilateral vocal cord are para-lyzed acutely by local anesthetic. Compare to Figure 7-6, which was taken at a more negative angle. Although SmF (facial canal) is easily located in this image, identification can be difficult when there are many surrounding mastoid air cells, especially in MRI. C is formed by the developmental fusion of the basiocciput with the basisphenoid, which are laterally separated by cartilage. This can give rise to the false impression of a skull base fracture on a lateral skull x-ray of an infant. The marrow cavity of the fused bone appears homogeneous on CT scan and in adults is filled with fatty marrow (see Figure 7-7). C is a frequent location for chordomas.

C	Clivus
CaF	Carotid Foramen
FM	Foramen Magnum
FO	Foramen Ovale
FSp	Foramen Spinosum
JF	Jugular Foramen
SmF	Stylomastoid Foramen

166 *Temporal Bone, Base of Skull, Cranial Nerves*

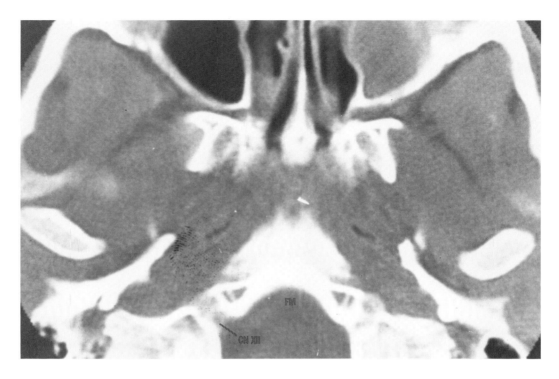

Figure 7-6 *Hypoglossal Canals*
CN XII passes through the anterior margin of FM and then continues into the hypoglossal canal. The occipital condyles are seen near the anterolateral margins of FM. CN XII is sometimes surgically anastomosed to the facial nerve below the skull base as a treatment for total permanent facial paralysis. Unilateral atrophy of the tongue will result, and the eyelids will close with tongue movements.

CN XII Hypoglossal Nerve
FM Foramen Magnum

CRANIAL NERVES

7-3-1 MRI: Sagittal

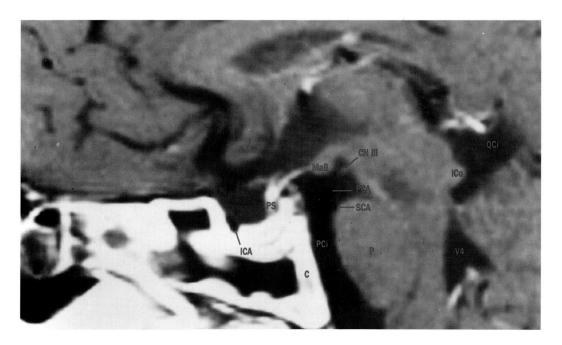

Figure 7-7 *T1-weighted, Oculomotor Nerve* The rootlets of CN III exit the midbrain on the medial aspect of the cerebral peduncles and course anteriorly through the interpeduncular cistern. The course of CN III then runs between PCA and SCA, more lateral than the plane of this section. After running parallel along the lateral side of the posterior communicating artery, CN III will then groove the lateral aspect of the posterior clinoid process before entering the roof of the cavernous sinus. CN III may be compressed by an aneurysm at the junction of the posterior communicating artery and ICA. ICA is seen within the cavernous sinus. The nucleus of CN IV is located in the midbrain at the level of ICo. CN IV exits the midbrain dorsally to decussate in the anterior medullary velum, in the roof of V4. C has intense signal because its embryonic red marrow has been replaced with fatty marrow during childhood. Partial replacement can give a zone of less intense signal and be confused with neoplasm (see Figure 7-5).

C	Clivus
CN III	Oculomotor Nerve
ICA	Internal Carotid Artery
ICo	Inferior Colliculus
MaB	Mamillary Body
P	Pons
PCA	Posterior Cerebral Artery
PCi	Pontine Cistern
PS	Pituitary Stalk
QCi	Quadrigeminal Plate Cistern
SCA	Superior Cerebellar Artery
V4	Fourth Ventricle

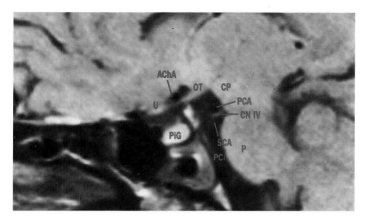

AChA	Anterior Choroidal Artery
CN IV	Trochlear Nerve
CP	Cerebral Peduncle
OT	Optic Tract
P	Pons
PCA	Posterior Cerebral Artery
PCi	Pontine Cistern
PiG	Pituitary Gland
SCA	Superior Cerebellar Artery
U	Uncus of Temporal Lobe

Figure 7-8 *T1-weighted, Trochlear Nerve* This image is 6 mm lateral to Figure 7-7. Having decussated through the anterior medullary velum (see Figure 5-9), CN IV curves around CP, passing through the ambient cistern. CN IV is seen here coursing between PCA and SCA within PCi. Thus, CN III and IV both run below PCA and above SCA. CN IV travels along the free edge of the tentorium, piercing the dura and entering the lateral wall of the cavernous sinus, below CN III. U is labeled at the point where it can herniate over the edge of the tentorium and compress CN III just proximal to its entry into the cavernous sinus.

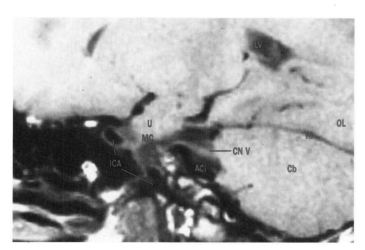

ACi	Ambient Cistern
Cb	Cerebellum
CN V	Trigeminal Nerve
ICA	Internal Carotid Artery
LV	Lateral Ventricle
MC	Meckel's Cave
OL	Occipital Lobe
TC	Tentorium Cerebelli
U	Uncus of Temporal Lobe

Figure 7-9 *T1-weighted, Trigeminal Nerve* This image is 9 mm lateral to Figure 7-8. CN V is the largest cranial nerve. It exits from the lateral aspect of the pons and passes through the lateral pontine cistern to MC, at the apex of the petrous portion of the temporal bone.

MC is a dura-lined structure containing cerebrospinal fluid and the trigeminal, or gasserian, ganglion. MC lies adjacent to the lateral wall of the cavernous sinus. ICA is seen at two points: inferiorly, within the carotid canal; and superiorly, exiting the cavernous sinus into the suprasellar cistern.

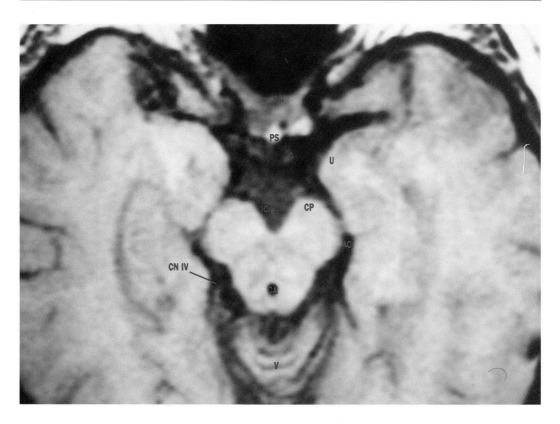

Figure 7-10 *T1-weighted, Trochlear Nerve* CN IV is seen here bilaterally within ACi. V is located below the fourth ventricle, where CN IV decussates. The course of CN IV continues around CP into the pontine cistern (see Figure 7-8).

ACi	Ambient Cistern
CA	Cerebral Aqueduct
CN IV	Trochlear Nerve
CP	Cerebral Peduncle
ICi	Interpeduncular Cistern
OC	Optic Chiasm
PS	Pituitary Stalk
U	Uncus of Temporal Lobe
V	Vermis of Cerebellum

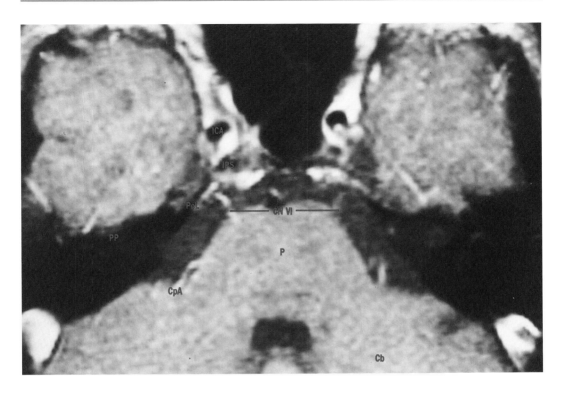

Figure 7-11 *T1-weighted, Abducens Nerve* CN VI is seen here bilaterally in this diabetic patient. CN VI on the right is enhanced with contrast because of microvascular disease. Note the lateral course of CN VI as it exits the pontine aspect of the pontomedullary junction. This is why CN VI is difficult to locate on a sagittal section. PP appears as the hypointense area lateral to CN VI. Inflammation of this bony structure, as in Gradenigo's syndrome or nasopharyngeal carcinoma, can cause CN VI palsy. CN VI pierces the dura of the posterior fossa to pass under PcL through Dorello's canal, where it is tethered and may be injured in conditions causing increased intracranial pressure. Tumors of the CpA region may extend to directly involve CN VI. They most commonly arise from the acoustic nerve either as an isolated tumor or as a part of neurofibromatosis type II. In addition to hearing loss and facial paralysis, they may exert pressure on the pons and produce a characteristic nystagmus, Brun's nystagmus with large-amplitude gaze paretic nystagmus on ipsilateral gaze and small-amplitude high-frequency nystagmus on contralateral gaze.

Cb	Cerebellum
CN VI	Abducens Nerve
CpA	Cerebellopontine Angle
ICA	Internal Carotid Artery
IPS	Inferior Petrosal Sinus
P	Pons
PcL	Petroclinoid Ligament
PP	Petrous Pyramid of Temporal Bone

Name _____

Address _____

City and State _____ Zip _____

Telephone (_____) _____ *Academy Member ID# _____
        area code

*Your ID Number is located following your name on any Academy mailing label, in your Membership Directory, and on your Monthly Statement of Account.

CATEGORY 1 CME CREDIT FORM

Ophthalmology Monographs 6

Magnetic Resonance Imaging and Computed Tomography: Clinical Neuro-Orbital Anatomy

You may claim 1 hour of Category 1 Continuing Education Credit, up to a 25-hour maximum, for each hour you spend studying this Ophthalmology Monograph. If you wish to claim continuing education credit for your study of this monograph, you must complete and return the self-study examination answer sheet on the back of this page, along with the following signed statement, to the Academy offices:

American Academy of Ophthalmology

P.O. Box 7424

San Francisco, CA 94120-7424

ATTN: Education Department

I hereby certify that I have spent _____ (up to 25) hours of study on the Ophthalmology Monograph *Magnetic Resonance Imaging and Computed Tomography: Clinical Neuro-Orbital Anatomy* and that I have completed the self-study examination. (The Academy *upon request* will send you a transcript of the credits listed on this form. You can check the box below if you wish credit verification now.)

☐ Please send credit verification now.

Signature _____ _____
                                              Date

MONOGRAPH COMPLETION FORM

Ophthalmology Monographs 6

Answer Sheet for
Magnetic Resonance Imaging and Computed Tomography:
Clinical Neuro-Orbital Anatomy

Question	Answer					Question	Answer				
1	a	b	c	d	e	15	a	b	c	d	e
2	a	b	c	d	e	16	a	b	c	d	e
3	a	b	c	d	e	17	a	b	c	d	e
4	a	b	c	d	e	18	a	b	c	d	e
5	a	b	c	d	e	19	a	b	c	d	e
6	a	b	c	d	e	20	a	b	c	d	e
7	a	b	c	d	e	21	a	b	c	d	e
8	a	b	c	d	e	22	a	b	c	d	e
9	a	b	c	d	e	23	a	b	c	d	e
10	a	b	c	d	e	24	a	b	c	d	e
11	a	b	c	d	e	25	a	b	c	d	e
12	a	b	c	d	e	26	a	b	c	d	e
13	a	b	c	d	e	27	a	b	c	d	e
14	a	b	c	d	e	28	a	b	c	d	e

SELF-STUDY EXAMINATION

The self-study examination for *Magnetic Resonance Imaging and Computed Tomography: Clinical Neuro-Orbital Anatomy* consists of 28 multiple-choice questions and is intended for use *following* completion of the monograph. Questions are constructed so that there is one "best" answer. For each question, record your initial impression on the answer sheet by circling the appropriate letter. It is recognized that a disagreement about the optimal answer may occur despite the attempt to avoid ambiguous selections. A discussion of the most appropriate answer to each question follows the examination. Answers should not be consulted until the entire examination has been completed.

QUESTIONS

1. CT is the optimal method for the initial acute study of all of the following conditions *except*

  a. proptosis

  b. head trauma

  c. unilateral abducens paresis with pain

  d. acute loss of consciousness

  e. painful, incomplete oculomotor palsy with pupil involvement

2. Contrast enhancement can be useful in all of the following situations *except*

  a. CT of orbit for lacrimal fossa mass

  b. T1-weighted MRI of suspected optic nerve meningioma

  c. T2-weighted MRI of suspected optic nerve meningioma

  d. fat-suppressed MRI of suspected optic neuritis

  e. CT of sella for bitemporal hemianopsia

3. MRI is preferred to CT in the initial evaluation of all of the following conditions *except*

  a. impaired elevation of one eye

  b. impaired elevation of both eyes

  c. downbeat nystagmus

  d. oculopalatal myoclonus

  e. long-standing bilateral superior oblique paralysis

4. A high-intensity signal will be seen in all of the following *except*

a. melanoma on a T1-weighted scan

b. perivascular tissue on a gadolinium-enhanced first-echo scan

c. fresh blood in the vitreous on a T1-weighted scan

d. ambient cistern cerebrospinal fluid on a second-echo scan

e. orbital fat on a first-echo scan

5. Reformatting of imaging data can provide all of the following advantages *except*

a. saves scan time with uncooperative patients

b. allows rotation of structure into multiple planes

c. localizes multiple orbital foreign bodies

d. provides information about thin structures in the origin plane of the section

e. allows retrospective analysis of data without the cost and inconvenience of repeating the scan

6. All of the following vascular problems would be well imaged by the technique listed *except*

a. midbrain arteriovenous malformation: CT with contrast enhancement

b. midbrain arteriovenous malformation: MRI T1-weighted, nonenhanced

c. dissecting aneurysm of the internal carotid artery: MRI T1-weighted, nonenhanced

d. aneurysm (> 1.0 cm) of suprasellar internal carotid artery: MRI angiogram

e. dissecting artery aneurysm of the internal carotid artery: CT with contrast enhancement

7. All of the following can be contraindications to gadolinium-enhanced MRI *except*

a. cochlear implants

b. cardiac pacemakers

c. stainless-steel–wired frontal process of zygoma

d. sickle cell anemia

e. severe claustrophobia

8. All of the following are attributes of the vidian canal *except*

a. conducts pericarotid sympathetic nerves

b. located in the sphenoid bone

c. superior and lateral to foramen rotundum

d. conducts the greater superficial petrosal nerves

e. when fractured, can lead to a dry eye

9. All of the following affect the MRI appearance of the optic nerve *except*

   a. chemical shift

   b. fat-suppression techniques

   c. first-echo imaging

   d. orbital as opposed to intracranial location

   e. T1-weighted as compared to T2-weighted imaging

10. The optic foramen could be well imaged on axial slices angulated so that it would include the

    a. lens

    b. internal carotid artery

    c. medial rectus muscle

    d. anterior clinoid process

    e. intraorbital optic nerve

11. All of the following statements are true *except*

    a. The radiofrequency bandwidth of the exciting pulse controls slice thickness.

    b. Pixel size is determined primarily by slice thickness.

    c. Short longitudinal relaxation times produce hyperintense signals on T1-weighted images.

    d. Long transverse relaxation times produce hyperintense signals on T2-weighted images.

    e. T1 is much longer than T2.

12. All of the following statements are true *except*

    a. Gray matter is much lighter than white matter on T2-weighted images.

    b. Saturation recovery is a fat-suppression technique.

    c. The letters TI on a film and the absence of fat signal indicate an inversion recovery (IR) sequence.

    d. T1 is an inherent tissue characteristic.

    e. T2-weighted scans have long TR values.

13. Optic nerve meningioma is visualized optimally by

a. axial CT scan of the orbit

b. coronal CT scan of the orbit

c. axial T1-weighted MRI scan of the orbit

d. coronal gadolinium-enhanced MRI scan of the orbit

e. coronal T2-weighted MRI scan of the orbit

14. The superior ophthalmic vein can be imaged in all of the following orientations *except*

a. longitudinal section, medial to the globe on coronal scan

b. cross-section, posterior and medial to the globe on axial scan

c. longitudinal section, posterior to the globe on axial scan

d. longitudinal section, anterior and superior to the globe on axial scan

e. cross-section, posterior to the globe on sagittal scan

15. T2-weighted MRI scans are most useful in showing

a. temporal lobe meningioma

b. thyroid ophthalmopathy

c. hydrocephalus

d. iron deposition in the basal ganglia

e. optic chiasm glioma

16. The trigeminal nerve is visualized in all of the following MRI scans *except*

a. axial scan through the pontine cistern

b. coronal scan through the foramen ovale

c. sagittal scan through Meckel's cave

d. axial scan through the midbrain

e. coronal scan through the optic chiasm

17. Which of the following statements about MR angiography is true?

a. It requires intravenous contrast agent.

b. It is obtained by having the computer subtract the dark signal from T2-weighted scans.

c. It is obtained by selectively imaging vessels with a predetermined flow velocity.

d. It is accurate in detecting orbital vascular anomalies.

e. It produces images as detailed as cerebral angiography.

18. The tumor that would be imaged optimally with CT is

a. choroidal melanoma

b. retinoblastoma

c. optic nerve glioma

d. basal cell carcinoma located at the medial canthus

e. orbital cavernous hemangioma

19. All of the following are appropriate angulations on an axial scan for the structure listed *except*

a. 0° for the pituitary gland

b. +20° for the foramen magnum

c. −20° for the optic foramen

d. −10° for the occipital cortex

e. −15° for the superior rectus muscle

20. T1-weighted scans normally show intermediate high signal in all of the following structures *except*

a. vitreous

b. cavernous sinus

c. sinus mucosa

d. pituitary stalk

e. posterior pituitary gland

21. All of the following statements about the nasolacrimal duct or bony nasolacrimal canal are true *except*

a. The inferior concha is a separate bone.

b. The superior and middle conchae are part of the ethmoid bone.

c. Conchae are seen on bone window CT scans.

d. Turbinates are imaged on MRI scans.

e. The structure extends superolaterally to inferomedially.

22. All of the following statements about the cribriform plate are true *except*

a. It is a part of the sphenoid bone.

b. It is a part of the ethmoid bone.

c. It can be fractured during dacryocystorhinostomy.

d. It passes branches of the olfactory nerves.

e. It is usually lower than the upper border of the medial rectus muscle.

23. After retrobulbar anesthesia, structures attached to and enclosed by the upper tendon of Lockwood can be invoked to explain all of the following consequences *except*

a. loss of adduction

b. loss of abduction

c. dilation of the pupil

d. sparing of depression and incyclotorsion

e. numbness of the tip of the nose

24. Proptosis is least likely to result from a congenital or acquired defect in which bone?

a. frontal

b. ethmoid

c. sphenoid

d. lacrimal

e. maxillary

25. The first-named structure is superior to the second-named structure in all of the following pairs *except*

  a. abducens nucleus, facial nucleus

  b. lingual gyrus, cuneus

  c. centrum semiovale, corona radiata

  d. internal cerebral vein, vein of Galen

  e. foramen rotundum, vidian canal

26. The second-named structure is one through which a nerve to the first-named structure passes in all of the following pairs *except*

  a. lacrimal gland, internal auditory canal

  b. Bowman's membrane, Meckel's cave

  c. lateral rectus muscle, petroclinoid ligament

  d. superior oblique muscle, prepontine cistern

  e. superior rectus muscle, upper tendon of Lockwood

27. Imaging which of the following structures is least likely to yield diagnostic information concerning optic nerve-head swelling?

  a. anterior clinoid processes

  b. periventricular white matter

  c. optic nerve sheaths

  d. petrous pyramid of temporal bone

  e. sella turcica

28. Abnormalities of the first-named structure can be imaged with the second-named disorder in all of the following pairs *except*

  a. posterior cerebral artery, unilateral pursuit deficit

  b. cerebellar tonsils, downbeat nystagmus

  c. nondominant hemisphere angular gyrus, agraphia

  d. agenesis of the corpus callosum, Aicardi's syndrome

  e. agenesis of the septum pellucidum, de Morsier's syndrome

ANSWERS AND DISCUSSION

These answers and explanations are to help you confirm that the reasoning you used in finding the most appropriate answer was correct. If you missed the question, the answer may help you to decide whether it was due to misinterpretation of the question or to poor wording. If, instead, you missed the question because of miscalculation or failure to recall relevant information, the answer and the explanation may help fix the principle in your memory.

1. **Answer—e.** While MRI scans are usually more definitive than CT scans, CT is preferred in most acute situations because of availability and short scan time. Surgical decisions can usually be made on the basis of the findings. If needed, MRI can be performed later. CT can define the anatomy, even if not the pathogenesis of proptosis. CT does not have the resolution to demonstrate aneurysms unless they are quite large and, therefore, MRI is often indicated to rule them out. Acute blood and acute infectious processes are best initially screened by CT because both processes are difficult to separate from high-signal fat on MRI without special techniques.

2. **Answer—c.** Because the relaxation-shortening properties of gadolinium are greater on T1-weighted scans, gadolinium is rarely used in T2-weighted imaging.

3. **Answer—a.** Because of artifacts induced by the skull base, CT images are inferior to MRI images of the brain stem. Response options b through e all represent lesions in the midbrain, pons, cerebellum, or medulla. Impaired elevation of one eye is usually orbital and, therefore, CT is an acceptable initial scan.

4. **Answer—c.** Fresh hemorrhage is dark on T1-weighted images. As the blood organizes in subacute and chronic stages, the center of the hemorrhage will become bright on T1-weighted images. Melanin contains free radicals and, therefore, exhibits paramagnetic characteristics. As a result, T1 and T2 are shortened, creating a bright signal on T1-weighted scans and a dark signal on T2-weighted scans. If the tumor is amelanotic, it will not create as dramatic a signal, but will still be brighter than vitreous on T1-weighted scans and darker than vitreous on T2-weighted scans. Fat has a short T1, which produces a high signal on a first-echo scan.

5. **Answer—d.** Reformatting data cannot increase the amount of information obtained in the plane of imaging. Spatial resolution can be improved only by decreasing the slice thickness of the sequence, decreasing the field of view, or increasing the acquisition matrix.

6. **Answer—e.** CT resolution is not good enough to detect the difference between the wall of the vessel and the dissection and cannot visualize the pathology as well as MRI.

7. **Answer—c.** The miniscule magnetic displacement induced in stainless-steel wires and microfixation plates used to repair bony fractures is insufficient to prevent MRI scanning. Cochlear implants can be dislodged, cardiac pacemakers may have their programs erased, claustrophobic patients can have severe attacks, and sickling can be induced by the strong magnetic field of the MRI scanner.

8. **Answer—c.** The vidian canal is medial and inferior to the foramen rotundum (see Figure 3-11).

9. **Answer—a.** Volume averaging plays a large role in the appearance of MRI images. A good example is the darker appearance of the optic nerve within the fat-filled orbit versus the relatively lighter appearance of the intracranial optic nerve and chiasm within the cerebrospinal fluid–filled crural fissure. Fat in the orbit adjacent to the nerve can alter the magnetic properties of the nerve itself; this is why fat-suppression techniques are so important in the orbit. Chemical shift artifacts create shadows alongside the nerve, affecting the appearance of the meningeal sheath, but not changing the appearance of the nerve itself.

10. **Answer—d.** The anterior clinoid process is located lateral to the optic foramen and posteromedial to the superior orbital fissure. Because the superior orbital fissure is 10 times the diameter of the optic foramen, a section that does not demonstrate the clinoid is likely to miss the foramen and show the much larger fissure only.

11. **Answer—b.** A pixel is a two-dimensional projection of the signal intensity and is independent of slice thickness, as distinguished from the voxel, which is a three-dimensional space.

12. **Answer—b.** Saturation recovery is a pulse sequence used to eliminate blood-flow and movement artifacts on T1-weighted scans.

13. **Answer—d.** T1-weighted MRI with gadolinium shows an intense bright signal in meningiomas due to strong enhancement. MRI scans performed without gadolinium are inferior to CT (which may show calcification) in the ability to detect and differentiate meningiomas. The coronal plate can demonstrate the tumor in the optic nerve sheath encircling the optic nerve.

14. **Answer—a.** The superior ophthalmic vein is seen only in cross-section on coronal scans. It can be seen in both cross-sectional and longitudinal planes on axial and sagittal sections.

15. **Answer—b.** The extraocular muscles are best contrasted from the orbital fat on T1-weighted images. T2-weighted images produce a bright signal from cerebrospinal fluid–containing spaces. As a result, they are useful in demonstrating dilation or compression of the ventricles. The low-signal edema associated with tumor is also seen. Iron deposition is prominent on T2-weighted scans due to iron's paramagnetic effect.

16. **Answer—a.** Because the trigeminal nerve is the largest of the cranial nerves, it is readily visualized in many MRI projections. It can be seen in Meckel's cave on coronal scans and on axial scans of the midbrain. On coronal scans, branches of the nerve can be recognized in the cavernous sinus and in the foramina ovale and rotundum. The portion of the nerve anterior and lateral to its exit from the base of the pons is not well visualized on axial scans through the pontine cistern.

17. **Answer—c.** MR angiography can selectively image large or medium-sized arteries by detecting flow rate and direction. In addition, cerebral veins and venous sinuses can also be viewed by this technique. Conventional angiography requires intravenous contrast. Computer subtractions are usually performed during digital subtraction fluoroscopic angiography studies to subtract the bony structures that are detected by conventional x-rays. Orbital vascular anomalies are most accurately depicted by conventional angiography. Cerebral angiography remains the ultimate standard as the most sensitive means of visualizing vascular anomalies and anatomy.

18. **Answer—b.** CT is superior to MRI in the detection of calcium; thus, CT is the preferred study in assessing bony structures as well as tumors that calcify, such as retinoblastoma.

19. **Answer—d.** Axial scans are sectioned in relation to the orbitomeatal line (OML). Orbits and optic canals are usually scanned at $-10°$ to $-30°$. Intracranial structures are most often imaged at $0°$ to $+25°$ with less positive angulation preferred for the sellar region, the middle range for the cerebral hemispheres, and the most positively angulated images for the posterior fossa. A scan performed at an inappropriate angulation may miss vital information.

20. **Answer—a.** Structures with a high fat content usually appear bright on T1-weighted images. Cerebrospinal fluid and vitreous appear dark because of their high water content. These structures are hyperintense on T2-weighted scans. Due to slow venous flow, the cavernous sinus and pituitary stalk have an intermediate signal on T1-weighted scans. Sinus mucosa usually has an intermediate signal on T1-weighted scans, but may have a high signal with inflammation.

21. **Answer—e.** The nasolacrimal duct or bony nasolacrimal canal extends superomedially to inferolaterally. Frequently, failed probings result from trying to push the probe toward the nose when, in fact, the bony nasolacrimal canal runs in the opposite direction.

22. **Answer—a.** The cribriform plate is a part of the ethmoid bone and is easily fractured during surgery involving the medial orbital wall. Coronal scans of the orbit reveal that it is frequently lower than the superior border of the medial rectus muscle.

23. **Answer—d.** The trochlear nerve passes through the superior orbital fissure outside the upper tendon of Lockwood that contributes to the annulus of Zinn. The nerve is thus outside the muscle cone and may not be anesthetized with a retrobulbar block.

24. **Answer—d.** All of the bones listed have more surface area in contact with the orbit than does the lacrimal bone, and all but the lacrimal bone contain a sinus cavity that can harbor a focus of inflammation or tumor that may decompress into the orbit.

25. **Answer—b.** The cuneus is the portion of the occipital lobe that is above the lingual gyrus, from which it is separated by the calcarine fissure.

26. **Answer—d.** The trochlear nerve arises from the dorsal aspect of the pontomesencephalic junction and, after decussation, passes through the ambient cistern, where it pierces the free border of the tentorium cerebelli behind and lateral to the posterior clinoid process. The trochlear nerve is never prepontine.

27. **Answer—d.** Only a large tumor at the petrous pyramid of the temporal bone is likely to cause sufficient increase in intracranial pressure to result in papilledema. Isolated thrombosis of the petrosal sinuses is also an unlikely cause of papilledema. The optic foramina are included in views of the anterior clinoid processes. High signal in the periventricular white matter would argue for a demyelinating or inflammatory cause for optic nervehead swelling, and a pituitary tumor within the sella turcica could cause papilledema.

28. **Answer—c.** Agraphia is a part of Gerstmann's syndrome, which also includes alexia, acalculia, and left–right confusion. It results from a lesion of the angular gyrus of the dominant hemisphere.

INDEX

NOTE: Anatomic structures are followed by their abbreviations. Plain type indicates that the subject is discussed, but not labeled. Boldface type indicates that the subject is labeled, whether discussed or not. For labeled structures, the plane of imaging is indicated by a letter following the figure number: *a* = axial, *c* = coronal, and *s* = sagittal.

MEDICAL COLLEGE OF PENNSYLVANIA
AND HAHNEMANN UNIVERSITY